PSYCHOTIC ART

ARBOR SCIENTIÆ
ARBOR VITÆ

Founded by C. K. Ogden

The International Library of Psychology

ABNORMAL AND CLINICAL PSYCHOLOGY
In 19 Volumes

PSYCHOTIC ART

FRANCIS REITMAN

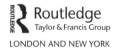

Routledge
Taylor & Francis Group

LONDON AND NEW YORK

First published in 1950 by
Routledge and Kegan Paul Ltd

Reprinted 1999, 2000, 2001 by
Routledge
2 Park Square, Milton Park, Abingdon, Oxfordshire OX14 4RN
711 Third Avenue, New York, NY 10017
Transferred to Digital Printing 2006

Routledge is an imprint of the Taylor & Francis Group, an informa business

First issued in paperback 2013

© 1950 Francis Reitman

British Library Cataloguing in Publication Data
A CIP catalogue record for this book
is available from the British Library

Psychotic Art
ISBN 13: 978-0-415-20933-5 (hbk)
ISBN 13: 978-0-415-86875-4 (pbk)
Abnormal and Clinical Psychology: 19 Volumes
ISBN 13: 978-0-415-21123-9
The International Library of Psychology: 204 Volumes
ISBN 13: 978-0-415-19132-6

CONTENTS

CONTENTS

v

ILLUSTRATIONS

FOREWORD

THE PSYCHIATRIST, by dealing with the total personality, tends to become a Jack-of-all trades; he measures his patients' body-configuration and their mental abilities; he assesses his patients' electro-encephalographic records and their paintings; he interferes with his patients' cerebral structure and with their set of values, and so forth. Furthermore, psychiatrists assume the right to generalize and give opinions on brain functions in general, on politics and sociology, on art and religion. These aspects, enumerated at random, require highly specialized knowledge, and psychiatrists cannot deal with them exhaustively; they can manipulate with them only in order to attempt some synthesis of their patients' personality. As to the generalization, this is only permissible if the psychiatrist maintains throughout that he does so from his own limited viewpoint.

With these tendencies and criticism of them in my mind I set out to examine psychotic art from one of the psychiatric viewpoints. Though necessarily this study is a psychiatric one, it was intended for interested non-psychiatric research workers as well, and in consequence the description of some phenomena had to be out of proportion to others.

On the other hand, problems in writing this study were created not only by the diversity of possible readers, but also by the diversity of the various approaches to be synthetized, such as neurology, psychometrics, psychology, sociology, aesthetics, etc. I had the advantage of co-operation from experts in these various fields, and had the help

of Mr. J. P. S. Robertson, who offered valuable criticism
and advised me on several relevant points. I wish to
express my gratitude to him and to others for their help,
viz. Dr. E. C. Dax for giving me facilities for this study
and permitting me the use of his case material; the Hon.
W. S. Maclay for advice and permission to publish some
pictures from his collection; to several of my colleagues
whose cases I investigated; to Mr. E. Adamson, art
therapist. I am grateful to Mr. Herbert Read and Mr.
Geoffrey Grigson for their encouragement. I would also
like to acknowledge the help of my secretary, Miss A. M.
Silkstone. I could not have completed this study without
the encouragement of my wife, to whom this book is
dedicated.

Sussex, 1950.

I

DEFINITIONS AND APPROACH

Employment of terms "psychotic" and "art" in the present study — Former studies of psychotic art — Art as a result of human cerebral function can be viewed biologically — Description of the present biological approach, termed the psycho-physiological.

I

THE PRESENT INQUIRY is concerned with the pictorial art of psychotics. Before this subject can be examined it is necessary to clarify one's terms, and in particular to discuss the sense in which the words "psychotic" and "art" will be employed.

The term "psychosis" will accord with the description of Henderson and Gillespie: they state that psychosis involves a change in the whole personality of the individual in whom it appears, his apprehension of reality changes qualitatively and his behaviour alters in consequence. So far as the various forms of psychosis are concerned, in this investigation the schizophrenias will feature predominantly; descriptions of this class of disorder, leading to a definition of it, will be given subsequently at a relevant point. The paintings and other artistic products of neurotics have been deliberately excluded from consideration here. The differences between neurotics and those conventionally called "normal" by some criterion or other are so finely graduated that a sharp delineation is almost impossible. If one judges neuroses by criteria that are purely sociological, it is possible to argue (as several writers have done) that creative artists in any medium are almost bound to be categorized as neurotic. Many investigators now consider that there is no sharp break at any point between the normal and the psychotic; instead there is a succession of graded differences from the normal through the neurotic and the severely neurotic to the psychotic. Even if one grants this proposition, the first and last categories are so far from each other on the scale of differences that they contrast sharply. Thus one can support a quantitative theory of psychosis and still be justified in dealing with psychotic art in contradistinction to normal art.

The concept "art" presents much greater difficulties and demands fuller discussion. This investigation is limited to "pictorial art", which is meant in most cases throughout the study (according to a common usage), whenever the term "art" is employed. Brief references, however, will be necessary to analogies presented by other forms of art and to art as a general concept irrespective of its medium.

The definition of art has always been elusive for art critics and art historians, aestheticians, philosophers and psychologists. Dictionaries define art in terms of a synonym "skill" or as "application of skill". While this corresponds to certain established usages it is too wide for aesthetic purposes. As a working hypothesis E. Newton defined art as "an original human conception, made manifest by the skilful use of a medium". Herbert Read in his earlier works seems largely to agree with this definition: as when he declared art to be "the technical skill" required "to transform mental images into linear signs". He added that the artist is capable of allowing "the personality to express itself in the craftsmanship". All such descriptions as these offer a useful point of departure for the art-historian who, having done with the definition, turns to his main subject; but they do not entirely clarify the meaning of "art". Read has developed the various approaches to art that have been developed to further our understanding of its nature. He has described genetic, metaphysical, aesthetic, phylogenetic, sociological and other approaches. These give information about the possible moral function of art, about the interrelation between art and society and about the motifs of artistic developments in savage communities, but they do not satisfactorily demarcate art from other human activities.

Read, in his important work *Education through Art*, to which further reference will be made, has added his own definition, which is in terms of receptive and expressive phenomena. According to this, art has two basic principles —the principle of *form*, which is a function of perception, and the principle of *organization*, which is a function of imagination. On the expressive side Read mentions "bodily action". The neuro-psychiatric objection to a formulation in these terms will be mentioned below. Here I need only say that the modern psycho-physiological conception of the working of the brain is contrary to the proposition that cerebral functions at the higher levels are receptive or expressive and hence ultimately reflex in nature. That Read's definition is based on the reflex character of functions at the higher levels is indicated by his description of the mind: "mind is like an automatic telephone exchange with senses ringing up every second asking to be connected in every direction", and "mind is the reservoir of all senses". Another shortcoming of Read's formulation lies in the principle of origination, which is explained by means of "imagination". For imagination, in turn, the hypothesis "the subconscious" is utilized. Thus the hypothesis of the definition rests on yet another hypothetical concept (see also Chapter 7). These objections are not aimed at criticizing the thesis to which Read's definition leads; they show only that such a definition does not allow the application of the technical tools of a psycho-physiological approach.

The problem stands thus: how are we to differentiate certain human activities, or the products of certain human activities which we call art, from all other human activities? In accordance with modern theories of definition and method, many difficulties can be avoided if we make our point of departure from the concrete and the readily verifiable and thence lead up to what is abstract and not easily confirmed. The theory developed in the following paragraphs has been suggested to me by Mr. J. P. S. Robertson.

The first verifiable fact with which we are concerned is that there are objects called paintings in art galleries, art exhibitions, on the walls of private houses and elsewhere. The overt activity by which these are produced may be observed by going to the studios of artists or by watching them at work in the open air. Activity of this kind has been going on for a number of centuries. The paintings are in the first place smears of paint on surfaces such as panel, canvas or paper. There are closely similar objects in which lines are drawn on surfaces with pen and ink, charcoal, or in many other ways, but everything that will be said of paintings can be applied to these with only slight modification; for simplicity the discussion will be confined at this stage to painting. The next verifiable fact is that these objects are not usually apprehended by the onlooker as smears of paint; the great majority of them by far make us think, or give us the semi-illusion, that we are seeing an actual situation (the difficulties raised by the term "actual situation" will be discussed shortly). This fact can be readily confirmed in particular instances: for example Chagall's "Sleeping Poet" in the Tate Gallery makes us think that we are looking at a man asleep in a field with farm buildings in the background, farm animals, trees and so on. It would be possible to value paintings according to the fidelity or accuracy with which they present this appearance of an actual situation which the spectator can perceive visually. Such a criterion is applied by many spectators at art galleries and art exhibitions, as anyone who listens to their comments will soon discover. It is not, however, the criterion applied by art critics or by those spectators who derive certain feelings of intense satisfaction from looking at the paintings. Nor do the painters themselves usually conform to any such system of valuation.

This leads to the next verifiable fact. These situations which the paintings make us think we are perceiving visually are deliberately "structured" in a way that actual situations in visual perception are not. Their relations have been ordered so that a pattern of form, shading and colour is produced. Consideration of painters at work indicates that this ordering into a pattern is usually a "re-structuring" of an actual situation visually perceived by the artist. The re-structuring is carried out by selection, rearrangement and qualitative alteration of form, shading and colour. Memories of other actual situations may be involved in various complex ways. The product may sometimes be based entirely on a re-structuring of remembered situations. Everything that has been said of painting is applicable to pictorial art in other media, such as pen-and-ink drawings, except that patterns of shading or colour may be absent in them. It must be noted that the re-structuring into a pattern is a phenomenon quite distinct from the fact that the perceived situation is represented in a two-dimensional and static medium, though it has a relation to it.

It is now possible to define pictorial art as a sub-class of pictorial products, the latter being defined ostensively. Pictorial products which are not pictorial art will be discussed shortly. Pictorial products can be called pictorial art when the situation which they make us think we are perceiving visually is structured into a deliberate pattern. This definition accords with the usual intention of the artists and the criteria by which modern art critics evaluate the art product; it is on the fact of structuring into a pattern that the feelings of satisfaction experienced by trained spectators depend when they view certain pictorial products. Differences in the effectiveness of the structuring constitute the scale of aesthetic values. The criteria by which these differences are judged show historical and geographical variation which will be discussed in a subsequent chapter. It is merely necessary to note here that art products differ in aesthetic value and that we are concerned, as so very often is the case, with a graded phenomenon. In the effectiveness with which the process of re-structuring is carried out there are two inter-related but separable kinds of skill: there is the executive skill involved in the manipulation of the medium and the intellectual skill involved in thinking out the pattern. This matter will also be discussed later on.

Besides differing in the effectiveness, according to certain criteria, with which they structure into a pattern the appearance or semi-illusion of an actual situation, paintings differ also in the extent to which a re-structuring has taken place. In some instances, notably in what is called "abstract" art, in the work of Cubist painters, in certain paintings of Picasso and others, the re-structuring is carried so far that the appearance or semi-illusion of viewing an actual situation is lost and the work becomes a pure study in design, in relations of form, shading and colour. While such work is certainly visual art, it is questionable whether it can still legitimately be termed "pictorial" art. In most cases, however high the degree of re-structuring, the appearance of an actual situation or some reference to perceived actuality is usually retained. The extent to which a variety of aesthetic satisfactions can be given by paintings which are pure design seems limited. Most spectators seem to need for their satisfaction this appearance of viewing an actual situation; and most "abstract" painters return periodically to some reference to actual perception in order that they may enrich and vary their performance. However that may be, it is certainly a fact that the great majority of paintings combine two characteristics: they give to the spectator the appearance, or semi-illusion, that he is beholding an actual situation, and they structure this situation into a pattern.

Paintings and drawings may contain a narrative component; they may tell or illustrate a story. An obvious example is Hogarth's "Marriage à la Mode". They may contain a propositional component: they may advance some contention or exhortation that could also be expressed in words. There are many examples of this in

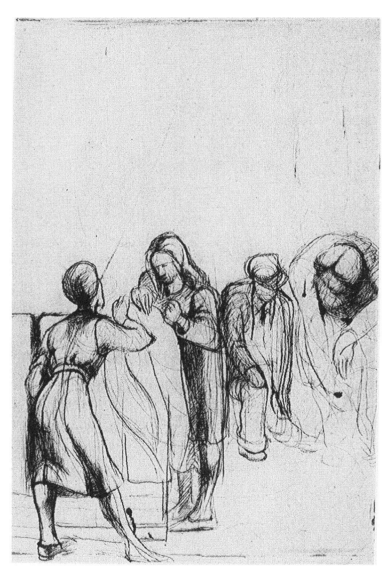

Fig. 1. 'A Most Important Composition'

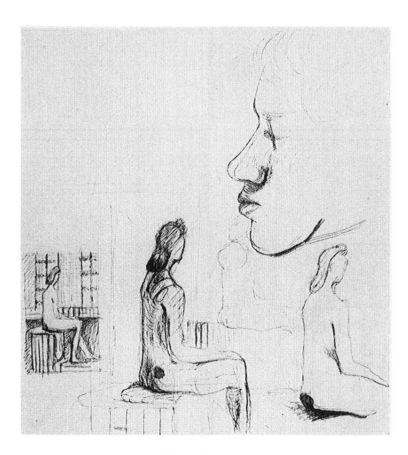

Fig. 2. Figures

poster painting—for instance, the war-time poster of a man with his hand on his lips to express what could be verbalized as "Be silent" or "Discretion is desirable". They may contain components that evoke feelings other than the aesthetic satisfaction arising from the pattern; they may depict a situation that arouses tenderness, pity, indignation, reverence, horror, disgust or other emotions. The subject depicted may have associations which are pleasurable in a particular cultural group, at a particular time or place; this applies to religious and erotic subjects, subjects having a mythological, historical or literary allusion, and so on. Other additional components are possible in paintings. But no such additional component— narrative, propositional, emotional, allusive or of any other kind—is either needed or enough to make a pictorial product into "pictorial art" as the term will be used in this inquiry. Such components are neither needed nor enough, because they do not in themselves arouse the feeling of satisfaction which is based on structuring into a pattern. Whether they actually impede the stimulation of such a feeling or diminish it, is an arguable question. It will be assumed here that they do not necessarily have these effects, but are variables completely independent of artistic value. This is not to deny that such matters of content in pictorial art are of great interest and importance and that the satisfaction from them may mingle in a complex way with the satisfaction arising from the structuring into a pattern of form, shading and colour. What is affirmed is that only the last-named characteristic is necessary and sufficient to make a pictorial product "pictorial art", as the term will be used in this study. Matters of content are, of course, especially important in psychotic paintings and will need to be examined in due course.

The description of situations as "actual" or "real" and the references to a process of the re-structuring of actuality raise certain difficulties where psychotics are involved. By an "actual" or "real" situation is meant what one visually perceives when one looks at houses, streets, people about their business, stretches of countryside, animals and so on. It is not necessary in an empirical investigation to consider metaphysical problems or to go beyond the assumptions of everyday life and biological science. Thus one ignores the question whether such perception gives true knowledge, and assumes that when two normal individuals look at the same object or situation their visual perception will be closely similar and for practical purposes may be considered the same. The difficulty arises in distinguishing aesthetic re-structuring of actuality from the re-structuring that occurs in the phantasies of normal individuals, both artistic and non-artistic, and from the qualitative alteration in the apprehension of reality that is taken as a defining characteristic of psychosis. So far as the phantasies of normal individuals are concerned—daydreams, night-dreams and allied processes—it is almost certainly true that they are composed entirely of elements from the remembered perceptual experience of the individual and that the remembered perceptual experience is re-structured in various ways, as a rule much more radically in the case of night-dreams than of day-dreams. This re-structuring differs from the re-structuring of art. First it is not expressed in a relatively permanent medium, and secondly (the important difference) it is usually a re-structuring of events in accordance with wishes and fears, and never a re-structuring into a pattern that accords with certain widely held criteria. When it is said that psychotics show an altered apprehension of reality, it means obviously that reality becomes re-structured for them. The psychotic re-structuring differs from the artistic re-structuring because it is not into a pattern that accords with certain criteria and because the psychotic accepts his re-structuring as being reality—which is one of the chief reasons why he finds his way into a mental hospital. The normal artist remains aware of reality as it is and knows that he has deliberately re-structured it in his art product. So does the spectator who looks at the product. The difference between the various ways of re-structuring have deliberately been formulated in the sharpest manner possible in order to show the general tendencies; in point of fact, the differences need not be so absolute, and there do exist intermediate states.

The subject-matter of pictorial art may derive wholly or partly from day-dreams and similar phantasies or from recollection of night-dreams. Surrealist painters acknowledge that night-dreams have given rise to many of their pictures; a similar source for other pictures may be inferred. All this is interesting as a matter of content and may give certain adventitious satisfactions to the spectator; but it is quite irrelevant to the status of the product as art, which still depends on the extent to which its pattern of form, shading and colour accords with the criteria by which art products are estimated. The extension of the subject-matter of pictorial art to such fields as night-dreams opens up, of course, many new possibilities of patterning.

One or two other points should be briefly mentioned in connection with reality and art. Sometimes it is argued that the artist "really sees" the situation as he paints it; this can be true only if "see" is used metaphorically. Some commentators would emphasize abstraction and selection from what is given in visual perception rather than re-arrangement and qualitative alteration of it; the evidence is strong that all these processes co-exist. In regard to reality, the appreciation of natural beauty—for example, of landscapes or mountains—is sometimes raised as a problem. This lies outside our scope, but it may be noted that such appreciation is probably for the most part consequent on the work of pictorial artists and other artists, such as poets, rather than antecedent to it.

The complex motivations that lead the normal artist to produce his work will not be directly considered in this inquiry, but they may be illuminated indirectly in dealing with the motivations that lead psychotic patients to produce paintings. At this point it can merely be left as an unanalysed fact that the artist finds great satisfaction in his achievement. The satisfaction found by trained spectators in their apprehension of the structuring of a pictorial art-product will also be left as an unanalysed fact; its biological history and sources will not be investigated. The structural relations that are necessary to produce it and the historical or geographical differences in regard to these, that is to say, historical or geographical differences in aesthetic criteria, will be given some consideration in the next chapter.

One should now refer briefly to art as a general concept. To ask, What is art as a general concept? is to ask, What have pictorial art, sculpture, architecture, music and literature in common?

Restriction of the term to these general media is purely arbitrary and many aestheticians would extend it much further, for example, to ceramics, the ballet, and so on. It is, however, historically true that up to the present most individuals capable of producing aesthetically satisfying work have chosen one of the five media named. These media at present offer to those trained to appreciate them the greatest possibilities of varied and intense aesthetic satisfactions. How far the limitation depends on biological, how far on sociological factors, will not be discussed here. If one disregards all the important differences between these five art-forms and asks what remains in common, one quickly sees that it is the structuring of perceptual material into a pattern which is satisfying by recognized criteria—in sculpture and architecture a pattern of three-dimensional form, in music a pattern of sound relations, in poetry usually a pattern of sounds and images, in prose literature a pattern of described human events or behaviour, and so on. In so far as products in any other media become art, it is because they are structured into a pattern. These remarks will be sufficient, for our purpose, to relate pictorial art to other forms of art.

How far to this concept of structuring into a pattern can the notion of "configuration" be applied? In recent years the term "Gestalt" or "configuration" has become the cloak for much loose and vague thinking and evasion of careful analysis. It is used to denote a number of distinct phenomena, all more or less involving the notion "wholeness" or "unity of parts". But how far is it true to say that a painting or other pictorial art-product must constitute a whole? Certainly a painting is a self-sufficient and self-contained system in relation to its actual surroundings, the frame, the wall, other paintings and so on. It is also true that the various relations constituting its pattern are usually all consonant with each other according to the criteria of art. In these senses a painting is a "whole". The subject-matter often, though not always, has a unity irrespective of the design, but the content is irrelevant to the status of the painting as art, in the way in which we have defined art. The relation of wholeness exists in the painting, but it is only one of many relations and it can easily be too much emphasized. In particular it is almost certainly wrong to argue that a painting can only be apprehended as a whole and still more wrong to say that it can be apprehended as a whole in one immediate swoop. All the testimony from artists and the aesthetically appreciative indicates that an artistically satisfactory painting has manifold relations in its structuring. Now one of these comes to the forefront of the spectator's awareness, now another. When he returns to the painting on a different occasion he is aware of still others. The relation of the whole is usually present only in the background of awareness as a schema. A similar contention applies to the effect of music, literature and the other arts. The facts seem to be best described by saying that a work of art is a more or less complex isolated system of relations of various kinds. If that is what is meant by a configuration, then a work of art is a configuration.

Pictorial art has already been related to other forms of art. It is desirable to relate it to pictorial products which are not art. The basic biological fact leading to all pictorial activity is that some objects make it appear to the spectator in a more or less illusory way that he is visually perceiving other objects. Such objects may occur naturally: they may be rocks, dead trees and clouds. They may also be produced by human activity in making smears or marks on a surface, which is the starting point of pictorial production. How and when early man discovered this fact and began to act upon it can be treated only speculatively. The drawings of young children explain the matter as little as their acquisition of speech explains the kindred problem of linguistic origins; children are born and grow up in communities where pictorial production is already an established, many-sided activity; the means of drawing are placed in their hands and they arrive at drawing with the encouragement and instruction of those about them. Once smears or marks make it appear that we are looking at other objects, we may develop in our picture-making in various directions. We may structure our representations into a pattern so that they become pictorial art. On the contrary we may make the representations more and more closely faithful to the appearance of the object or situation which they resemble. Pictorial products then become a tool of practical and scientific activities; examples are anatomical or botanical drawings. In this development the skills of close observation of what is drawn and effective manipulation of the medium are involved; the more complex skill of thinking out a pattern is absent. How far this development has now been rendered obsolete by photographic techniques is a debatable question. Another development is in the direction of schematization so that the product finally ceases to be a representation; this leads to diagrams, alphabets, conventional signs and so on. A quite different development is that of expressing or communicating situations which the individual cannot, or for some reason does not wish to, verbalize—situations he fears or desires. This is an especially important development with psychotic patients and must be dealt with more fully as the study proceeds. Products of this kind may or may not be pictorial art according to the presence or absence of deliberate structuring. Such a motivation may sometimes be present in the work of normal artists, but consideration of exhibited works suggests that it is very uncommon. The foregoing remarks will be sufficient to establish the status of pictorial art in relation to other pictorial products. Once again the distinctions have been made sharp for the sake of clarity; once again there are intermediate possibilities. The important fact is that, while pictorial art-products may be valued as aesthetically satisfying or not in various degrees, there are pictorial products which are neither good art nor bad art by any criteria—they are not art at all.

This leads to the problem of how far pictorial art and other pictorial products may be regarded as symbols. The theory of signs and symbols is complicated and has many aspects; the terms "sign" and "symbol" are employed by various writers in different ways. There is general agreement that an object may be termed a sign or symbol if it is attended to not for its own sake but for the sake of something else to which it refers. In pure cognition one may follow G. F. Stout in differentiating *expressive* signs which are attended to through a series of activities with continuous reference to what they signify, *suggestive* signs in which attention immediately passes from the sign to what is signified, and *substitute* signs which are attended to through a series of activities with reference to what is signified only at the beginning and end of the process. Examples of expressive signs are words, of suggestive signs traffic lights, and of substitute signs most mathematical symbols. When orectic and sociological factors are taken into account many other classes of sign or symbol may be distinguished. There are symbols used for concealment except from the initiated, such as codes; symbols used to denote occupational class, such as uniforms, or relative status, such as badges of rank; symbols designed not only to denote group membership but to promote group solidarity, for example flags and political emblems; symbols used allusively to evoke feelings or for pure ornamentation, of which there are religious or literary examples. There are also the Freudian dream symbols, which, in so far as they are a fact, may be regarded as a variety of the symbols used for concealment, the concealment being from the dreamer himself. Sometimes objects are attended to partly for their own sake and partly with symbolic reference. There are many further ramifications in the theory of signs and symbols with which we need not be concerned. The question is, at what points do pictorial products fit into the schema we have outlined?

As the smears and marks on a surface are not attended to for their own sake, pictorial products might be subsumed under the class of signs and symbols. They differ, however, from all the varieties of symbol we have considered in that they make it appear to us that we are perceiving the object or situation to which they refer. This difference is so great that it seems best not to treat them as symbols but to class them as a different phenomenon, as "representations", just as stage-plays are representations. Only when the component of representation is quite lost while at the same time external reference remains, as in diagrams, do pictorial products develop into real signs of the expressive variety. Another important point must be noted. Pictorial art products *are* attended to for their own sake so far as the essential structuring into a pattern is concerned; they may be said to combine two aspects— an external reference to what they represent and an intrinsic value as a structuring into a pattern. When pictorial art products develop into art products that are pure design they lose all exterior reference and are attended to entirely for their own sake. For these reasons it seems inappropriate to call pictorial art *per se* symbolic. It is another matter that the content of pictorial art may sometimes be wholly or in part deliberately symbolic in that objects depicted may signify something other than themselves. An obvious example is afforded by the objects in Holbein's "Ambassadors". This may occur for ornamentation and evocativeness, or because the painting advances some proposition. Anyway, it is a matter of content and neither necessary nor enough to make the painting art, within our definition. Such deliberate symbolization, however, is of some importance, as we shall see, in discussing the pictorial products of psychotics, especially those which express or communicate what the patient cannot verbalize.

A number of writers have argued that the subjects or

situations depicted by artists have a symbolic meaning for them of which they are unaware, either of the sexua Freudian or the mystical Jungian variety. Leaving this for a time, it may be said that while such unconscious symbolization may perhaps have been satisfactorily demonstrated in particular normal or abnormal painters, its general occurrence has never been empirically shown and *a priori* is exceedingly improbable.

The use of the terms "psychotic" and "art" has now been elucidated. Psychotic patients make pictorial products, some, but not all, of which are pictorial art. In so far as such products are pictorial art they may be estimated and enjoyed in precisely the same way as the productions of normal artists. The methods of patterning, however that are chosen by psychotics are of special interest in connexion both with the theory of psychosis and the theory of art. The content or subject-matter of psychotic pictorial products is irrelevant to their status as art but is of great intrinsic interest in relation to general psychology and in relation to the theory of psychosis. Before coming to the special characteristics of psychotics both in patterning and in subject-matter, it remains in the second section of this first chapter to describe previous work in the study of psychotic pictorial activities, to discuss in general the applicability of scientific method to aesthetic questions, and to set out in particular what is meant bv the psycho-physiological approach.

II

The subject of "psychotic art" has been admirably reviewed by Anastasi and Foley (1940) and an extensive survey of the literature on it up to 1946 is given in the works of Pappenheim and Kris. The various approaches to psychotic art have been grouped by Maclay and Guttmann into three categories. *First* the clinical approach, which attempts to ascertain how far his psychotic drawings are typical (symptomatic) of the mental disease of the patient. Such studies were the outcome of the static psychiatric theories originated by Kraepelin. With the introduction of dynamic concepts into psychiatry, the interest was focused on parallels between personality changes and stylistic alterations. Experimental work utilizing this approach began as far back as 1906, when Mohr attempted to investigate the personality structure of schizophrenics by letting them copy figures. Similar techniques were reported by me in 1939, leading to the conclusion that psychotics, especially schizophrenics, fail to appreciate and are unable to reproduce facial expression in drawings; sometimes only the latter incapacity is evident. The *second* category of approach in the study of psychotic drawings is the psychological one; these methods have been dynamic and interpretative and ultimately speculative about the genesis of pictorial art. The most outstanding psychological work is that of Prinzhorn, who studied the art products and life-histories of psychotics, correlated them, and attempted general conclusions on the nature of art. His explanations, however, such as "the universal urge for expression . . . manifested in form tendencies" are merely substitutes for such concepts as "inspiration", and they fail to answer the genetic problems of art. Furthermore, Prinzhorn maintained that ethical values are essential factors in psychotherapy and he introduced such valuation when assessing the art products of his patients; he thus became frankly subjective. The last factor leads us to the *third* category of approach to psychotic art: the aesthetic approach, that of some psychiatrists, who have attempted to compare psychotic art with recent developments in non-psychotic painting.

What, we have to ask at this point, is the relationship of scientific to aesthetic valuation? A value may be regarded as a fundamental dimension of differences. In a crude form it is a dichotomous classification: in ethical valuation into good and bad, in scientific valuation into true and false, in aesthetic valuation into artistically satisfying and artistically unsatisfying. In its more developed form valuation is graded and relativist; in ethical valuation actions become more or less desirable according to certain principles or standards; in scientific valuation theories become more or less credible as approximations to the truth, in aesthetic valuation products become more or less artistically satisfying. In both the crude and the developed forms scientific and aesthetic valuation are basically different dimensions. Scientific valuation rests on the "quite-so" feeling of conviction; aesthetic valuation rests on the satisfaction produced by apprehension of structuring into a pattern. The sharp difference is shown by the fact that scientific products such as Newton's Theory of Light are rated as more or less probable in the existing state of knowledge, but aesthetic products such as Botticelli's "Birth of Venus" or Beethoven's "Emperor Concerto" have no relation to probability whatsoever. A scientific valuation can be altered by the adducing of fresh facts or consideration; aesthetic valuations do not alter in this way at all—they alter when for historical and sociological reasons there are changes in the criteria by which a patterning is judged to be artistically satisfying. If, then, the two dimensions are fundamentally different, how can aesthetic products be studied scientifically? The answer is that in the last analysis one cannot produce scientifically the feeling of aesthetic satisfaction in those that do not experience it, nor can one adduce reasons why an individual ought to prefer one set of aesthetic criteria to another. In the same way we cannot in the last analysis adduce reasons why people should be humanitarian or prefer one ethical code to another. One can, however, attempt to study scientifically the biological origins of the feeling of aesthetic satisfaction. One can study how far the criteria of aesthetic value are biological and innate, how far they are sociological and acquired. One can also attempt to correlate differences and changes in aesthetic valuation with cultural and social differences or changes. The aims of this book are more modest than that. They are to study the special characteristics in form and content of psychotic pictorial activity and to investigate its motivation. A psychiatric estimation of art thus aims to remain a scientific approach and must concern itself with truth only. Below, I shall inquire into problems of psychotic art from a psychiatric standpoint. I shall examine data collected hitherto, and criticize them. I shall attempt to show the biologically determined dynamics of this human characteristic: art. "Biologically determined dynamics", however, is a phrase which calls for more detailed description, all the more as this is my own basic attitude in treating the material.

The specific characteristics of man distinguishing him from the sub-human species lie in his capacity of conceptual thinking. This capacity enabled man to alter and re-create his environment, to create in general, and, *inter alia*, to create art. The capacity of conceptual thinking is basically related to the brain. Here some explanations are necessary. The mental functions have been for long looked upon as reflex in their nature, having been conveniently subdivided into receptive and expressive functions. It was imagined that an initiation from outside, that is to say, a sensory stimulus, arrives at the brain, is relayed and delayed, initiating an expressive phenomenon which is manifested in motor action. Thus the cortical cells were looked upon as a kind of inter-nuncial (connector) system and their functional entirety was imagined to rest upon an afferent and efferent branch of a reflex arc. Sherrington, however, clearly refuted this out-moded conception of mental functions in his Gifford lectures, when he argued that the cortical cells of the roof brain act spontaneously and not as a result of sensory activation. He rightly pointed out, that as the cells of the stomach do not rest between meals but prepare themselves for the next feeding time, similarly the cortical cells remain active even during sleep. They are, as Sherrington emphasized, self-activating. Support for this comes from electro-encephalographic (E.E.G.) studies; these have shown that the so-called "alpha waves" are, as Gray Walter termed them, inaction potentials; they are records of cellular activities in rest, *without* an initiation from outside. Sleep also has a typical E.E.G. record, and is not an abolition of the waves. These findings support Sherrington's thesis, that the cortex is a self-activating structure; hence cortical function should be assessed on a different basis from that of the reflex phenomenon. Thus the study of psychotic art on a neuro-physiological basis must, since psychotic art is a phenomenon of dysfunction, be related in some way to the brain. Upon that level cerebral physiology needs to be considered in terms of psychology and psychiatry, in other words, psychiatry and psychology must be, physiologically, the technical tools of our approach.

To give an example, Greek is a conglomerate of sounds which is perceived as such, if you cannot speak the language; but the same conglomerate of sounds becomes meaningful if you do speak that language. This does not mean that the physiological processes in the second example are different, but that they become broadened and integrated in such a way that they have to be assessed on the highest cerebral physiological level. To continue the analogy or verbalization, an aphasic disturbance (inability to speak or to understand speech without damage to the motor or sensory system proper) might be comparable with psychotic art. Aphasias are dysfunctions on the highest physiological level, and the analysis of these dysfunctions helped greatly to the understanding of the physiologica functions of speech. Upon this analogy one might ask: could not the analysis of psychotic art, viewed as a dysfunction, throw light on the physiological, namely, on non-psychotic art?

It was said that the technical tools of assessment on a high physiological level were psychiatry and psychology. The next problem arising is this: through what psychiatric approach should the results we obtain be assessed? In studying brain functions and mental life three types of approaches have been developed. First the neuro-psychiatric approach, which correlates mental life with cerebral structure; second, the psychosomatic approach, which interrelates structural and psychological factors as correspondent to each other; and thirdly, the psycho-physiological, which correlates mind and mental life not to structure but to the function of that structure. Head instanced the psycho-physiological views on walking, which is a group function. Now a lesion anywhere localized disturbs the smoothness of this combined function, resulting in an alteration of the function as a whole. Thus Head not only stressed the correlation of dysfunction to function, but also the significance of group function, the wholeness of function, and that a dysfunction should not be correlated to structure but to the original function of that structure.

To sum up: art is a mental manifestation based on human cerebral function. Such a conception allows formulation in such a manner that the problems can be assessed in terms of functions, that is, physiologically or else psychiatrically and psychologically. This might lead to recognition of biologically determined factors in psychotic art: if then the findings are related to function and not to structure of the brain, one might, to a limited extent, generalize from the psychotic to the non-psychotic art.

II

FORM IN PSYCHOTIC ART

The formal elements of schizophrenic paintings—The rôle of colour—Tendency to ornamentation—Mescalin drawings and the schizophrenic type of "doodle".

I

IN THIS CHAPTER, certain formal elements of psychotic paintings, and schizophrenic paintings in particular, will be examined. The early studies recognized that a painting by a manic-depressive, for instance, reflects the patient's excitement, in wild choice of colour, and in restless, disordered, incoherent lines. Mild depressives choose sombre colours; their pictures exhibit in their themes the poverty of their ideas. Severely depressed patients do not produce pictures at all, because of the inhibitory effect of their illness. Drawings of patients suffering from general paralysis of the insane are ataxic, vulgar and deteriorate to childishness. Senile drawings exemplify the ataxia of the patients; epileptics are the most willing dilettantes with a great gusto for pedantic detail. But, in general, it has been found that the total of paintings from all other groups of mental disease does not equal the wealth of painting produced by schizophrenic patients. The reason for this, which I shall discuss eventually, has been investigated by later workers. At present, as I have said, I shall deal only with the formal elements of schizophrenic paintings, though the subdivision is artificial, necessitating a reference from the one aspect of form to the other aspect of content.

Schizophrenic reactivity may be insidious in onset or it may take an acute form. A wide variety of schizophrenic symptoms may then be manifested. There may be extreme confusion of thinking and turmoil of emotion. These may be accompanied by states of perplexity or fear. The patient may exist in a state akin to that of a dream. He may show the phenomena called "dissociative"—his personality disintegrates into unconnected separate systems. He often exhibits "ideas of reference"; he believes that quite extraneous events have a special application to himself or that people are talking about him. These symptoms usually appear suddenly, often without any apparent precipitating stress. Inquiry, however, generally reveals historical evidence of preliminary symptoms. The acute schizophrenic reactivity is often accompanied by a pronounced effective tincture of either excitement or depression. The symptoms frequently clear up in a matter of weeks, but there is a tendency for them to recur. The schizophrenic reaction may pass into a chronic form in which varying mixtures of symptoms are exhibited.

Many of the various subtypes of schizophrenia have hallucinations of hearing as one of the typical symptoms; and the pictorial reproduction of hallucinations is a frequent characteristic of schizophrenic art. Visual hallucinations may also be elaborated pictorially and some examples of such work readily convey to the physician the ghastliness of hallucinatory experience. On the other hand, in the rapidly progressing types of schizophrenia the personality disintegrates and so do the artistic products, as one would expect. Such a rapid deterioration is well illustrated in Figs. 1–3. The patient had been an art-student before her illness began: her first drawing is technically skilful, but as a picture, meaningless. It is lacking in composition and the figures are merely pieced together without having any connexion with one another. The patient wanted to do "an important composition", but when asked what the picture meant she was unable

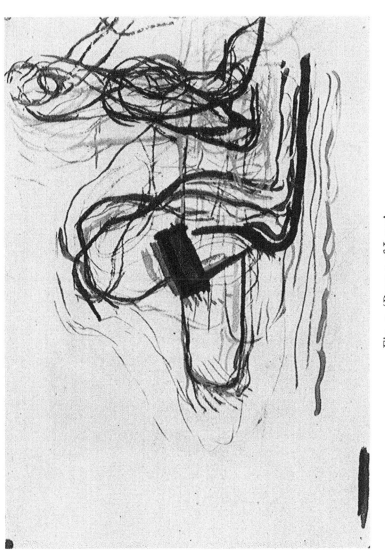

Fig. 3. 'Prayer of Love'

face p. 22

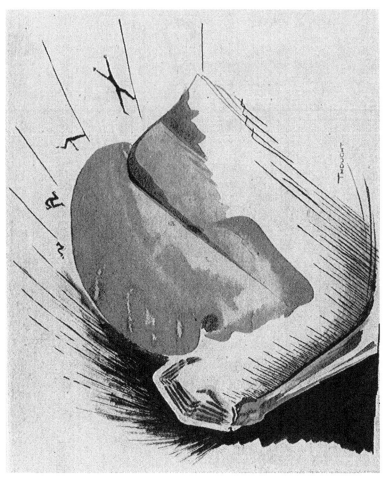

Fig. 4. 'Thought'

to say; she could not even give a title to it. This is not a frequent occurrence in schizophrenics, since they seldom become alienated from their own work. The second picture, painted a couple of months later, completely lacks any cohesion or composition; technically it is inferior to the first one, hardly indicating that its creator was an artist. The third picture was the last one she painted; at one time she called it "Prayer of Love", a bizarre expression without meaning—at least in relation to the picture itself. The outline of some figures can still be detected in the drawing, but it demonstrates that not only content but technique has deteriorated. The personality of the patient became fragmented and so did her drawings. The three paintings chosen as landmarks in the history of her illness were selected from a larger set of pictures; it should be mentioned that between the second and third pictures she created a few "ornamental" drawings. These are not reproduced because the progressive disintegration of her personality is better demonstrated by the paintings depicting figures.

Schizophrenic behaviour is unpredictable, and is often characterized by stereotypy, actions monotonously repeated by perseveration, repetition of an action after a stimulus, by mannerisms and bizarre actions. Such behaviour disturbances may first be "complex-determined" in the Freudian phrase, but become later a habit, from which meaning has completely departed. Those symptoms are readily detectable in schizophrenic paintings. One patient painted cubes in the same arrangement (in one corner of the sheet of paper) all the time. The cubes were always open. The meaning of this for the patient lay in its expression of the fact that a cube, though well defined towards the surrounding space, becomes absorbed in this surrounding space by being left open. In a few years this meaning disappeared and he kept on drawing the pictures in a mechanical and stereotyped way. Yet another patient used to start on a picture and then at one point, like a broken gramophone record, he would go on and on repeating the same motif in the picture (perseveration).

3

Bizarre reactions are expressed in the choice of content as well as in the style of the picture; such bizarre reactivity is shown in the next three reproductions (Figs. 4–6). They are paintings of a young man, who, before his admission, did not paint at all; he had no knowledge of pictorial art or of painters. He had never been to an exhibition and had never seen any work of "modern" art. This patient suffered from a schizophrenic type of thought disturbance and from bouts of depersonalization, that is to say, of sudden losses of belief in his own existence, an experience suggesting that he is no longer himself. Sometimes this experience was accompanied by the feeling that his surroundings were dream-like, distant and not real (de-realization). Fig. 4 is the first picture he painted, and he called it "Thought"; according to him the picture is self-explanatory. The development of a thought is shown as a fragment of a pensive black figure, which successively becomes more complete and ultimately flies away into space. The pensive figure originates from the big skull; it has no head, as if to illustrate that it is part of that skull. At this point it is not only the bizarre notion to which attention must be drawn, but the dominance of symbols as well. The hypertrophy or enlargement of symbols is a usual phenomenon in schizophrenic paintings, and psychiatrists have explained it in terms of schizophrenic thought disturbances. It has been said, that in schizo-phrenic thinking the symbol becomes identical with the meaning and is then experienced as the meaning. In other words, it is a kind of short-circuiting between con-cepts and their "concretistic" equivalents. More will be said about this later; here an example should suffice to illustrate what is meant. A patient of mine thought that as a private in the Army he had a dog's life; whilst on parade he suddenly went on all fours and started bark-ing. This was the manifest outbreak of his schizophrenia. In his disordered thinking, instead of "I am treated *like* a dog", he thought in a concretistic way, "I *am* a dog", and acted accordingly. To return to the picture; a thought arising *in* the skull is actually experienced as a fact arising *from* the skull. This is not an abstract symbolization of the knowledge that it arose as a cerebral function within the body; it is a concrete mode of thinking. Hypertrophy of symbols will be detected in several other schizophrenic paintings reproduced in this study.

The second picture produced by the patient was "The Man Goes over the Hill" (Fig. 5). Each hill stands for a stage in the man's life on which he leaves his mark; this is symbolically represented by his shadow, and in the foreground the rest of his shadow is visible. The shadow is flanked by two classical pillars, which are symbolic of the man's past. This picture in its structure is well balanced and well delineated in relation to the surrounding space; the system of patterning as a whole is pleasing and so is the choice of colour.

The third picture (Fig. 6) is less satisfactory, when compared with "Thought" or "The Man Goes over the Hill". It is not well balanced, its spatial organization is disturbing, and so is its system of relations as a whole. Its choice of colour is strikingly displeasing; here one should point to the curious effects in the painting of the use of red, as for instance the red which contrasts with the blue of the stairs in the foreground. Such red effects are favoured by schizophrenics, a fact to which W. S. Maclay drew my attention. It will be convenient now to discuss the rôle of colour in schizophrenic painting.

Schizophrenic patients, especially those who are chronic or deteriorated, are much bolder in their use of colour than normal individuals. Besides this, an unpleasing choice of colour is fairly typical of schizophrenic paintings in general. This is manifest in various ways. One aspect is a preference for colours not often employed by the normal and distasteful to them, such as the curious tone of red already described and certain other tones. Another aspect is seen in unsatisfactory interrelationships of colours, seldom favoured by normals. A third aspect is a tendency to depict objects in colours markedly at variance with those they possess in real perception. Empirical investigations into the colour-behaviour of schizophrenics have been chiefly concerned with their passive preference for colours and their relative tendency to react to form or to colour; there has been little experimental work to elucidate their active use of colour in painting. So any tentative explanations must be largely hypothetical.

It may be that in schizophrenic painting there exists a schism of a kind between form and colour; colour is employed as an element quite independently of form. This in turn may depend upon a disintegration of conceptual categories in relation to the outer environment. Again the schizophrenic treatment of colour may be a return to more primitive modes of reaction. A quite different possibility is that the schizophrenic has a special affective relation to particular colours and uses them merely because of their intrinsic appeal to him. Or the schizophrenic may feel a need to modify the colours of his environment in the most radical way that he can. Still another possibility is that parallel with the disintegration of the personality in schizophrenia the technique involved in painting the colour of light deteriorates; this would apply principally to changes in the use of colour by trained artists who have become schizophrenic. Evidence from diverse sources supports each possibility.

The responses of deteriorated schizophrenics to the Rorschach Ink Blot tests, in which coloured blots are used instead of blots of plain ink upon white, show a heightened reactivity to colour together with an inability to integrate the blots (which is the point of the test) into meaningful shapes. This would favour the possibility that in schizophrenic painting colour is divorced from form on the basis of a dissolution of clear-cut concepts about the external world. The evidence of the Rorschach test also supports the possibility of a special emotional relation to particular colours.

In brain lesions perception of form may be impaired or lost while perception of colour remains normal. Schilder described a case of carbon-monoxide poisoning where the patient was suffering from visual agnosia or inadequacy of perception, but his perception of colour he retained almost intact. I. Wechsler observed a similar case. These findings show the relative independence of the two perceptive functions and suggest that possibly in the schizophrenic process perception of form becomes weakened while perception of colour becomes heightened and at the same time modified by its separation from form.

Von Senden's studies of congenitally blind patients cured by operation indicate that colour is often perceived before form after vision is acquired. This fact hints that perception of colour may be more primitive than perception of form. The evidence, however, from the animal series and from child development is fairly conclusive that perception of form is the more basic and biologically the more important function. It seems that in the normal individual reactivity to colour is slight in very early childhood, rises rapidly to a peak in middle childhood, and diminishes steadily from adolescence onwards. It may be that the colour preferences and reactions of schizophrenics are a regression to those of middle childhood.

For the normal individual, in conceiving and manipulating his environment, categories of form predominate, categories of colour are definitely subordinate. In other words, our orientation towards our environment is dependent on sorting out shapes and attributing colour to them rather than *vice versa*. Schizophrenia is marked by a disintegration of categories in relation to the outer environment; one effect of this may well be the divorce of colour from shape. On the other hand, Goldstein found that schizophrenics tend to group shapes not by abstract criteria, but on an anthropomorphic basis, by attributing to them human qualities and relationships; perhaps schizophrenics in a similar way attribute human qualities to colours also and their odd colour-behaviour springs from such an attitude.

As for the disintegration of technique, treating the matter on the executive side, one must remember that a painter has to learn to see the colour of light instead of the colour of objects; he has to learn to see "picture colours". D. Katz has emphasized the part colour, or more particularly illumination, plays in the structuring of a work of art. If there are no special colour differences to distinguish the illumination within the picture from that outside it, the opposition between picture and reality disappears. "True art", adds Katz, "never seeks to destroy the dividing line between what is presented and what is real." Thus the painter who has become schizophrenic may *refuse* to work with "picture colours" and may revert to "object colours" as a consequence of his altered relation to reality (see Chapter 3).

The altered relation to reality leads to attempts of various sorts to reverse presented situations in some way. Examples are well-known in schizophrenic symptomatology; for instance, one schizophrenic insisted on beginning his dinner with coffee, then having his sweet, then meat and then soup. This reaction is specifically shown in regard to colour in response to the Kohs Block Design test. Schizophrenics sometimes arrange the blocks in a correct design with the colours changed or reversed. Schizophrenic painting of objects in colours markedly at variance with their colours in real perception may be due to a similar reactivity.

All these possibilities still need to be verified. Furthermore, the cerebral basis of colour perception is far from being settled, though it appears that fibres transmitting specific colour vision are ultimately relayed to the calcarine cortex, where the receptive, analytic part of colour vision ends. There is every reason to suppose that a synthesis of impulses is elaborated in neighbouring centres, but there is no record of an isolated disturbance of cortical colour synthesis. The patients investigated by Kleist and Pötzl who suffered from colour agnosia were also word-blind and thus fundamentally aphasic. Gelb and Goldstein relate colour agnosia to amnesic aphasic disturbances and evaluate it as a failure in categorical thinking. Thus, owing to lack of psycho-pathological and neuro-physiological studies, no further discussion is possible, but the importance of colour disturbances is considerable and attention must be drawn to them when the formal elements of schizophrenic paintings are considered.

It should be noted that the trained artist is essentially relational in his approach to colour in his painting, whether he formulates this clearly in a verbal statement or is only half-aware of it in an unverbalized way. This may be well illustrated by a quotation from Matisse. He describes his process of painting in the following manner: "If, on a clean canvas, I put at intervals patches of blue, green and red, with every touch that I put on, each of those previously laid on loses in importance. Say I have to paint an interior; I see before me a wardrobe. It gives me a vivid sensation of red; I put on the canvas the particular red that satisfies me. A relation is now established between this red and the paleness of the canvas. When I put on besides a green, and also a yellow to represent the floor, between this green and the yellow and the colour of the canvas there will be still further relations. But these different tones diminish one another. It is necessary that the different tones I use be balanced in such a way that they do not destroy one another. To secure that, I have to put my ideas in order; the relationships between tones must be instituted in such a way that they are built up instead of being knocked down. A new *combination* of colours will succeed the first one and will give the wholeness of my conception."* Similar accounts of the painter's approach to form have been given by Braque and Metzinger, to mention only two of modern artists. Clearly, the impairment of conceptual thinking in the schizophrenic patient makes it difficult or impossible for him to apply such a relational approach either to colour or to form.

The patient who created the painting in Fig. 6 wished to solve the problem of the "Reversal of Perspective" which is the title he gave to the picture. He indicated that the reversal of perspective is "the philosopher's problem", and that he is going to solve it pictorially, by lines and colour, and by a human figure, with a child's feet, to indicate the reversal of accustomed visual relations. When

* From *Notes d'un Peintre*, published in 1908.

his picture was completed he announced with satisfaction that "the problem is solved ". The picture presents a man whose head is up in the sky and whose feet are in the foreground; though one would expect the shapes in the foreground to be larger, the proportions are in the reversed direction. This same reversal is emphasized in the steps, which narrow as they approach the onlooker and contrast with some very large steps, to reinforce the effect. Similarly, the most disturbing factor in the picture, the white road and the reversedly smaller trees flanking it, emphasize the inverted proportions of the perspective. The red and green lines of the background give the picture a more restless effect.

The choice of such bizarre content might legitimately suggest that it reflects his own difficulties, and that the distorted body, in a disordered spatial relation, is a reflection of his feelings of depersonalization and derealization. In other words, the picture might express his distorted experiences of his own body. Moreover, it raises the important question of whether the underlying factors in schizophrenic depersonalization and derealization are primarily experienced in distortion of the body or in distortion of the spatial surroundings. To this problem I shall return. It seems to be significant that at first glance this third painting appears to be the worst: we experience in it an inverted configuration or system of relations. It is not the new or unexpected re-structuring of reality which disturbs us, but its destructiveness. This destruction is not only achieved through linear representations but through colour as well.

The bad configuration of the picture "Reversal of Perspective" we must consider at more length chiefly to clarify the sense in which the term configuration or "gestaltung" is used. Visual reduplication is a subdivision of space and corresponds to rhythm in music, which is a subdivision of time. Both are the most elementary factors in art, elementary because their relationship to the physiological is nearest. The pictorial artist brings elementary visual reduplications into relationships of varying degrees of complexity. He begins with a vague concept or schema of his picture and organizes the various reduplications into a pattern of relations to each other. If configuration or "gestaltung" is taken to mean this process of organization or its result, then it involves conceptual activity to a great degree. In schizophrenics a conceptual deterioration takes place and the organization of pattern disintegrates. The picture loses its unity and gives the impression of a bad configuration or a discordant system of relations. This phenomenon is also illustrated in the series of pictures of a cat reproduced in the frontispiece and Fig. 7. In the former, though ornamentation predominates, the picture is well organized as a whole; the cat's paw, its eyes, nose and ears, and the filling up of the space between them organize the factors in a pleasing unity. Fig. 7, however, does not show any organization; the cat is lost in a maze of parts. The picture has no delineation in relation to the surrounding space; if it were twice the size it would demand still more space. It is not a "restructuring", because it possesses virtually no structure. The parts do not hold together; what has taken place can be described as a refragmentation. Thus instead of configuration, "structuring" seems a more satisfactory term; the part colour plays in structuring has already been mentioned.

Spearman has drawn attention to the confusingly double meaning of this concept of "configuration". He emphasized that configuration not only concerns objective form, but also denotes a subjective grouping; the latter signifies the manner in which the form is regarded. Structuring, on the other hand, denotes a frankly conceptual activity or its product. The principles of this activity may be ascertained empirically, but it does not necessarily depend on any *a priori* laws of "gestalt". As McDougall pointed out, the laws of configuration can be easily fitted to facts which were known beforehand, but they are unsatisfactory means to use for prediction of unknown facts. Throughout the present study, the term "configuration" will always be used to denote conceptual activity or its product; for instance, when it is said that the body image is a *gestalt* or a configuration, this refers to its conceptual component. It is intended to denote a grouping and elaboration of various sensory impulses into a system of relations.

But to return to the frontispiece, the picture might also illustrate other points raised in the first chapter, such as the schizophrenic apprehension of reality. A "modern" artist's reconstruction might be unexpected, might appeal only to a few, whose perceptual and conceptual training allows them to follow the artist's problem and its solution; but the schizophrenic "reconstruction" is rejected, not merely unappreciated, because his "reality" is a distorted, an abnormal one. It can be estimated psychiatrically, but hardly appreciated aesthetically.

Mannerisms are often expressed in so far that alien elements may appear suddenly in the picture, which are not inter-connected in any way with its form or content. Alternatively, they may be expressed in a needlessly over-elaborated picture, often filling in every square millimetre of the available space. It seems that to such over-elaboration and ornamental stylization abstract forms lend themselves more suitably than attempts at representation. Indeed, pattern of form frequently predominates in schizophrenic paintings and the tendency to produce geometric forms instead of representative ones may accord with the alteration of reality for schizophrenics. Stylization as a result of the altered experience of reality in schizophrenics was first emphasized by adherents of the psychoanalytical school. They considered it to be a result of changed logical activity owing to emotional causes, and looked upon it as a magic means of altering and influencing reality. The principles governing stylization have been well summarized by Kretschmer. They are: emphasis of the essentials, simplification and the repetition of forms; the latter is achieved by bilateral symmetry and by multiplication of a single pattern.

It has been shown, however, that there is a strong physiological element responsible for the appearance of the ornamental in schizophrenic paintings. Kanner's experiments on optic imagery indicate a tendency to multiplication of the image itself. "The tendency to multiply perception is probably a primitive tendency connected with the optic-perception as such, which finds increased expression in optic imagination". Thus there seems to be a tendency to spontaneous multiplication of the images. The investigations of Kluever also support these observations: he studied the process of reproducing eidetic images and found fragmentation of the images, which at times are cut to pieces. Schilder argued that the mechanisms of this fragmentation are based on primitive optic experiences, in which simplified figures (spirals, waves and vortices) are important. Bender also observed that after injury to the brain complex figures revert to more primitive levels, and that again simplified patterns and reduplications make their appearance. These observations suggest a perceptual conditioning for stylization. However, the use of simplified patterns on more primitive levels, such as follows after injury to the brain, strongly supports the theory of the phylogenetic development of artistic configuration. Visual reduplication or repetition, as already stated, is the subdivision of space, just as rhythm is the subdivision of time. Both are the simplest forms of configurational activities; they are phylogenetically the first to appear in artistic creations, and when deterioration takes place they are the last to disappear. Stereotyped repetitions often accompany disintegration ot the central nervous system, as in senility, following encephalitis, etc. Thus it seems that the appearance of a strong stylistic element in the sense of excessive ornamentation in the art products of a patient indicates that he is deteriorating. Schilder and Levine, on the other hand, investigated geometric patterns in drawings, from a psycho-pathological point of view. Patients who were receiving group treatment were encouraged to draw. When "primitive, instinctual drives" became evident in the course of the group analysis, geometric stylization showed in the drawings of the patients. This group analysis was conducted entirely on psycho-analytic lines, and since they are related in terminology and evaluation exclusively to the Freudian school of thought, it is difficult to generalize from Schilder and Levine's conclusions.

The two pictures reproduced in Figs. 7 and 8, which have already been discussed in connection with the problems of configuration, also illustrate in dynamic fashion the tendency to stylization. They were painted by a professional artist who was ill; the choice of theme, the stereotyped cat, may be "complex determined", but this matters little in relation to the questions raised in this chapter. Before his illness, this artist's drawings of cats—impressionistic studies of cat's heads—were well known. I have not reproduced any of these more normal drawings. But as his illness gradually progressed, so his style altered, and as the years went by he tended more and more to ornamentalization. In the end he produced an over-elaborated, bizarre, ornamental pattern, which suggests a cat at all only in connection with the earlier drawings.

Support for the theory of a close link between perceptual reduplications and optic imagery comes from experiments with mescalin. Mescalin is an alkaloid produced from a Mexican plant; the natives of Mexico used it for its intoxicating effects and attributed demoniacal and supernatural powers to it. Experiments since the early nineteenth century have confirmed that mescalin produces a toxic state, accompanied by a transient mental derangement, not unlike schizophrenia. The experience itself is partly characterized by visual hallucinations of a very pleasant character, which change like the patterns of a kaleidoscope. No other drugs such as hashish or marihuana, induce visual hallucinations which are so intense. The drug is excreted through the urinary system within 24 hours. In some cases there is a slight after-affect accompanied by inco-ordination (ataxia).

The power of this drug to induce a transient schizophrenia-like psychosis has been utilized by several psychiatrists, some of whom have taken mescalin themselves to be able to judge of the experience personally. I myself, when I was under mescalin, was fully aware of my surroundings, but I asked people irritably to leave me in peace, so that I could enjoy my hallucinations undisturbed. This increased introspective tendency is one of the characteristics of mescalin experience, and more will be said about it in Chapter 3 in dealing with schizophrenic disturbance of thought. Let us confine ourselves at the moment to the visual effects. Maclay studied the mescalin hallucinations of subjects able to draw. He asked them to sketch their hallucinations instead of giving a verbal account of them. They appeared fleeting in shape, position and colour, and all the shapes tended to elongation and reduplication. Reduplicated zig-zag lines were frequent. Another fairly common character of the visual hallucinations was a "tapestry pattern". Knauer and Maloney's subjects reported mosaics and ornaments, spiral and windmill and carpet patterns; other workers have found that colour in mescalin hallucinations becomes dissociated from form. When Maclay studied the drawings of his subjects, he observed that the "tapestry" pattern was probably the reproduction of the choroid or intermediate coat of the subject's eyeball which was perceived and then painted. Fig. 8 is a painting by one of Maclay's mescalin subjects, representing the choroid in an artistic elaboration. Fig. 9 is an interesting parallel. This picture was painted by a schizophrenic patient under the following conditions: she was gazing out of the window absentmindedly, when she started to sketch the background, and the flower pot was elaborated later. Probably she experienced her choroid as an after-sensation and incorporated it into the picture which, with some phantasy, represents her two eyes and her nose. The point to emphasize, however, in both examples is the strongly physiological perceptual impetus which moulds the "artistic" expression. Maclay speculated on the psychological *versus* the physiological theories of hallucinations and concluded that at least in mescalin the hallucinations are physiological in origin, but that their content is determined psychologically.

Most probably, all experiences of the kind are interwoven in a similar way. *The examples reproduced were chosen to show the interrelation between perceptual pattern and optic imagery.* In an artistic sense the same interrelation was consciously utilized by Leonardo, who remarked that when contemplating a damp spot one may see chimeras and other phantastic figures in it: "this method of looking at fortuitous shapes may stir the mind to inventing things and can be, therefore, of importance for creative work. . . . it is a good education for the fancy".

One of the early symptoms of schizophrenia is the alteration of verbal expression. There seem to be odd sequences and inconsequences of ideas; associations seem to be directed by alliteration, instead of logical relationships. Speech becomes incoherent, fragmented and apparently meaningless. Various words are condensed into new words (neologisms): "convertical", "needies", are examples of the neologisms used by a patient of whom a fuller account is given in Chapter 4. But ultimately the lack of logical relationships, the quantity of neologisms, etc., make schizophrenic language unintelligible. Such nonsense language ("word salad") in schizophrenics sounds like a proposition, but it is not. It has speech value, by its perceptual merit only. Thus, actually it becomes a substitute for a communication: as Noyes puts it, it is a "self-meaningful" communication, which amounts to the same thing—it is no real communication at all. This tendency of words to lose their true content value and retain only a perceptual existence exemplifies the schizophrenic tendency to "perceptual" or "concretistic" thinking. As a result, a schizophrenic communication becomes a mixture of conceptual and perceptual factors; of pictures and words; of "self-meaningful" symbols and meaningful concepts. Such are—for want of a better expression—the schizophrenic "doodles". Several psychiatrists look upon such doodles as being primarily pictorial propositions mixed with "writing in" or the naming of what is drawn, the latter being a schizophrenic symptom. It is, however, futile to search for the primary factor in these products. As far as doodles have a meaning, they have it only in being a unity of drawing and writing; the lack of one of these components destroys the whole meaning or "self-meaning" of the doodle.

Before attempting further analysis of this schizophrenic type of doodle, some remarks on non-schizophrenic doodles seem to be necessary. Maclay and his collaborators studied doodles sampled from the "normal" population. They defined them as "graphic results of playful activity done without purpose, in a state of divided and/or diminished attention". They found that out of 500 specimens only 139 were devoid of "writing in". In form, these doodles exhibited stereotypy, ornamental details, movements, figures, faces and animals; they depicted scenes, medley, "mixtures" and ornaments. Maclay concluded that as far as the uniformity of doodles goes, they express physiological and psychological uniformity of human reactions. Though noticing similarities between doodles and certain schizophrenic drawings, Maclay carefully avoided any conclusions based on analogies alone. Doodles, he emphasized, are not communications and their meaning is only apparent in individual analysis; thus again they are only "self-meaningful". In this respect they have the most intimate relationship with the schizophrenic "doodle", described in this chapter.

Nonsense poetry is an artistic elaboration of verbal doodling; actually it is, as in the schizophrenic doodles, always a mixture of writing and drawing, both being closely interrelated, and only in conjunction making a proposition of some kind. The classical example of this is Edward Lear's nonsense. Carroll's nonsense is probably a conscious imitation of such doodling, of neologisms, etc. How far nonsense poetry is symptomatological is a speculation not within the problems of this present chapter. Enough is said if it is recalled that both the authors named have been subject to the curiosity of psychiatrists and that schizoid inclinations have been noted in each of them.

In considering the schizophrenic type of doodle, Fig. 10 should now be examined more closely. The circumstances in which the patient came to draw it were these: she possessed a copy book and pencils and after one of her former doodles had been seen she was encouraged to go on drawing. Thus she was not doing it as a message or for some purpose, but merely as a playful activity for no ulterior reason at all. The picture has no content and the patient's explanations, so far as she was capable of these, were a secondary paraphrase. Because of the meaninglessness or purposelessness of the picture, I am inclined to classify it as a doodling type of drawing. Its creator is a schizophrenic woman 30 years of age, with much disintegration of personality. Her illness was chronic and did not seem to respond to treatment. Only a few remarks from her explanatory attempts are given here. First, she remarked on the fact that she was related to an Earl of Shrewsbury. Then she emphasized that the picture should be viewed as history repeating itself. She drew attention to the centre of the composite figure. On the top of the picture are stars, and a key of hope. The central figure is "a man in woman, the woman in man". The fingers are Finland; this is evident just as much as Warsaw means "saw war". There are two lips on the figure which are tulips; Denmark is shaped geographically like a tulip. So, for instance, from the "past time" came Palestine. The picture is in a way a plan of the universe, and a plan of the globe. She also explained that the top figure is the male, God the Father; the duplication of this figure is God the Son and the female means three in one. She reverted to geographical explanations. There are three fatherlands in the drawing, Japan, China and Indonesia. Indonesia comes from the Danes, Daniel in the lion's den. Religion and Denmark stand for a "father-country". Then she turned the picture upside down. There is a female figure now. Her umbilicus is a cherub; the umbilicus is the navel, which is nose. Then the tubes are there, and the two lips which are the chamber of the womb. The writings on the picture denote the evil spirit of conduct being set aside for 3,000 years. The key of love is: hope. She went on in the same manner, "explaining"

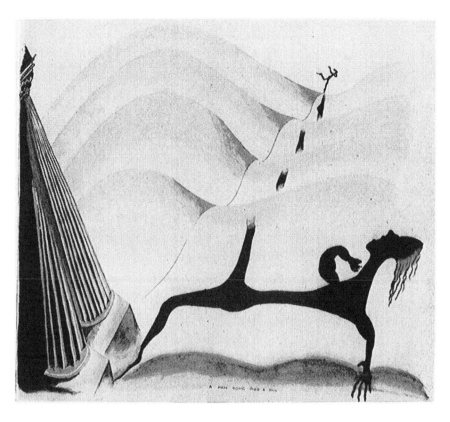

Fig. 5. 'A Man Going Over a Hill'

face p. 38

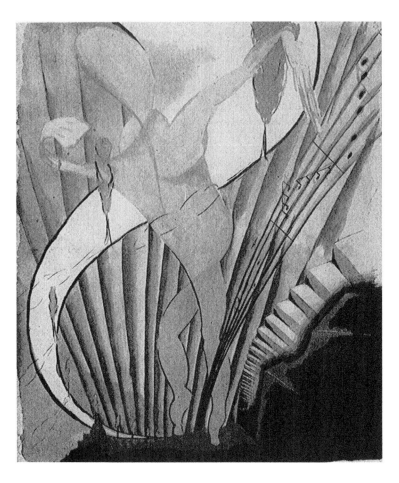

Fig. 6. 'The Reversal of Perspective'

the picture. All her explanations are illustrative of a "word salad" and of the schizophrenic type of association on a perceptual basis. They also illustrate the conceptual (structural) weakening shown in sentence formation. They really do not explain the drawing.

The composite figure in the picture is not dissimilar to neologisms: it is condensed from various parts, just as neologisms are formed from various words. In the same way as neologisms, such pictorial condensations are self-meaningful, comprehensible, that is, to the patients alone. Fig. 16, one of Goya's engravings, exhibits such pictorial condensation elaborated artistically; but as a picture it is also self-meaningful only. Among "modern" works, Picasso's "Minotauromachia" illustrates the same phenomenon, re-emphasizing the pictorial condensation with an artificial neologism. The psychoanalytical school has given much thought to the underlying mechanisms of such pictorial condensation, all the more as similarities have been found in them to dream mechanisms. Moreover, because of similarities between such drawings, and those of totemistic civilizations, conclusions have been drawn on the basis of superficial appearance—a characteristic heritage of nineteenth-century psychiatric reasoning.

It also deserves mention that several details of Fig. 10 refer evidentially to sex and many more would invite a psychoanalytical interpretation. Some of the sexual representations in the picture are almost obscene, a not infrequent feature of schizophrenic drawings. On the other hand, the appearance of Father, God, "the Woman in the Man", etc., are pleasing pictorial expressions of Jungian concepts. I shall come later to ask whether the Freudian and Jungian symbols are valid; but here, we seem to have a striking pictorial illustration of the *relativity* of such interpretative approaches.

Yet another type of "composite figure" often found in schizophrenic drawings is the Cephalopode. The appearance of such figures in children's drawings, amongst others, is probably indicative of the child's incomplete orientation towards his own body. I found that several of

4

my schizophrenic painters were motivated in a similar way, and I shall have more to say about this, mentioning here only one of my patients, who had greatly disturbed notions about the trunk of his body, which he wrapped up day and night in cotton-wool. In his drawings, not only Cephalopodes, but their symbolic equivalents appeared repeatedly; for instance, Humpty-Dumpty, or kites which possess head and tail but no trunk.

II

The various formal factors I have enumerated are not exhaustive; there are several others which have been left out and there may be still others which have not, as yet, been recognized. The presence or absence of one of these characteristics, however, does not alter the "diagnosis" of a schizophrenic picture. Such a diagnosis can only be made in any event, if one compares a series of pictures from the same patient, that is to say, if one views these pictures dynamically. Alternatively, one may relate the pictures to the patient and correlate the two together. Decisive, therefore, are the mental mechanisms behind the picture: it is which of these will determine whether one should view a picture as schizophrenic or not. No "diagnosis" can be made by studying one isolated painting.

III

THE CONTENT OF PSYCHOTIC ART

The schizophrenic reactions; their similarities to psychological dynamics in "primitives"—Disturbed ego demarcations of schizophrenics—The body image; its neurological and psychological aspects; its relation to schizophrenia.

THE PROBLEM THAT I now intend to examine is why schizophrenics are almost the only contributors to psychotic art. This entails an inquiry into the motivations impelling schizophrenics to paint.

First of all we must state the grounds of behaviour on which a patient is regarded as schizophrenic. In recent usage "schizophrenic illness" has been taken to represent a group of psychotic disorders characterized by fundamental disturbance in the relationship of the patient to reality and in his conceptual thinking or "concept-formation". These basic disturbances lead to further affective and intellectual disturbances in varying degrees and mixtures. The disorders are marked by a strong tendency to retreat from reality and by emotional disharmony. There are unpredictable interferences from within the patient with the sequence of his expressed thought. His emotional expression inclines to be "flattened out". His conative behaviour, in particular his reaction to biological drives, inclines to be altered. All these changes give an appearance of deterioration. The expectation that the patient will deteriorate still further may not be fulfilled. But he may progress to a stage of childishness called "schizophrenic dementia".

Important diagnostic evidence of schizophrenic reactivity, especially of disordered conceptual or "categoric" thinking, is afforded by special tests such as the Rorschach Ink Blots; the Vigotsky classification test and developments from it such as the Hanfman–Kasanin test; the sorting tests of Goldstein–Scherer, Rapaport and Halstead; tests based on proverbs and problems like those of Benjamin and Cameron; and Murray's Thematic Apperception test. The use of some such tests will be described more specifically in the next chapter, and the whole problem of conceptual thinking and its experimental investigation will be discussed in Chapter 5.

Schizophrenic reactivity may occur in a mild form which is revealed only by special procedures such as the tests I have named. Such cases rarely need admission to a mental hospital. The reactivity may, however, take an acute form.

The fundamental symptoms, then, in the schizophrenic process may best be regarded as the schizophrenic's peculiar ways of thinking or thought disturbances. His world seems organized into categories of time, space and logical relation quite different from those of the world of the normal individual. This is more evident as the illness progresses but the beginnings of the phenomenon can be detected in the earlier stages. Cameron found when he applied problem-tests and sorting tests to schizophrenics that they exhibited an allied phenomenon of "overinclusion"; they could not eliminate from the problem environmental and imaginal material only remotely related to it. Another allied phenomenon, occurring in everyday talk but particularly elicited by special tests, is that of contamination, a form of that condensation already discussed. Two separate notions occur simultaneously to the patient and he fuses them incongruously into one. A pin-man drawing was shown to a schizophrenic patient.

It seemed to her like a rope and also like a man; thereupon she described it as a "man-rope".

Besides the disturbances of thinking the other important feature of the schizophrenic reaction is an apparently complete apathy or loss of emotional response. Frequently also the patient seems "ambivalent" in his emotions; he expresses contradictory feelings, say love or hate, towards the same person or object, and these appear either to co-exist or to alternate very rapidly. This attitude occurs in the normal man, but to nothing like the same degree.

A resemblance has been argued between the thinking of schizophrenics and the thinking of pre-literate peoples, particularly by the French school of sociologists founded by Durkheim. These views have been particularly developed by Lévy-Bruhl in relation to primitive peoples. He has described the thinking of primitive tribes as "pre-logical" and accounts in these terms for such phenomena as magical practices and beliefs. The concepts of the primitive are vague, incoherent and ill-defined. The well-known notion of *mana* is a good example of such an ill-defined concept. Primitives are held not to proceed rationally from premise to conclusion but to jump illicitly and impressionistically in a manner similar to that which Piaget, in the field of child-psychology, calls "transductive reasoning". Resemblance is taken to mean identity. A person or object can be regarded as being simultaneously two different things: thus a leopard may be both a leopard and a man at one and the same time. This Lévy-Bruhl calls duality. Conversely they regard it as possible for one and the same person or thing to be in two different places at the same time; a man may be lying asleep and simultaneously may be hunting a hundred miles away. Lévy-Bruhl's term for this is bi-presence. Everything is looked upon as homogeneous in essence—people, animals, plants and stones. The boundaries of the self are not clearly defined. Most especially the real unit is the group, not the individual, as it is in advanced communities. A physiological, almost organic, solidarity exists between members of the same social group; individuality is almost completely submerged in this solidarity. The boundaries of the self are weak also in relation to component parts and property. The individual's secretions, excretions, footprints, the remains of his food, the objects he makes or handles, his personal property, his reflection or shadow—all are regarded as the man himself. It is this attitude that makes possible the practices of sympathetic magic. The resemblance between such notions ascribed to primitive men and some of the disorders in the thought of schizophrenics already described will be quickly apparent.

The psycho-analysts, notably Freud himself, Roheim and Money-Kyrle, have developed allied but somewhat different theories about primitive psychology which would also resemble schizophrenic reactions. They state that at an early period in cultural development the emotional life predominates over logical thinking; things or events are interconnected by their emotional importance, not their spatial or temporal coincidence. This emotional life of fears and desires is characterized by ambivalence, here taken to mean contradictory feelings towards the same object; these may be reverence and horror, or, as with schizophrenics, love and hate. The conflicting emotional experiences are apprehended as "good" and "bad" respectively, have to be accepted or rejected; they are projected outwards and constitute the basis of the notion of tabu, its sanctions, the constructs of demons and spirits and all the beliefs of animism. Such a system of emotional thinking Bleuler termed "dereistic"; it is also called "magic thinking". The practice of magic itself, according to this school of writers, is an attempt to resolve ambivalence of feeling by apparently meaningless behaviour, either active as in the development of rituals or passive as in the use of amulets. The apparently meaningless behaviour symbolizes the rejected part of the ambivalent feelings and leaves the savage free to experience the aspect that he wishes to accept. Money-Kyrle develops this theory further by considering magical fluids and substances (of which he regards *mana* as an example) to be projections outside the self of the body fluids and substances such as breath, urine or excrement; he treats supernatural creatures as similar projections outside the self of parts of the human body, for example, the breasts, the nipple or the penis, which are apprehended as either "good" or "bad" objects, or ambivalently as both.

The theories of the psycho-analysts are, to say the least, highly speculative. The views of Lévy-Bruhl and the French sociologists have also not found much favour with anthropologists working in the field. Anthropological objections were ably summarized by F. C. Bartlett some twenty-five years ago in a series of arguments which still remain valid. He notes that much of Lévy-Bruhl's evidence rests upon the "traveller's tales" of missionaries and traders rather than upon the observations of the trained investigator. Pre-logical thinking, he points out, is incompatible with the practical inventiveness of primitive man in the search for food, the provision of dwellings, and the development of material arts, crafts and techniques; all the evidence obtained in the field indicates that in such activities the pre-literate employ the same psychological processes of learning and reasoning as civilized man. This criticism would also apply to the theories of the predominance of emotional thinking, advanced by the psycho-analysts. Bartlett remarks that even in the realms chiefly dealt with by Lévy-Bruhl—those of death, disease, dreams, omens, wounds, war, desire and the like—pre-logical thinking is not absolute; Lévy-Bruhl's own illustrations contain examples where logical thinking is evident. Moreover, Lévy-Bruhl has made an antithesis not between the primitive man and the ordinary member of a modern social group but between primitive man and the scientific expert. Pre-logical thinking in the form of relating surprising and sudden events to remote and recondite agencies can be observed by anyone who cares to look for it in modern life almost any day he wishes; Lévy-Bruhl has almost completely neglected to observe the modern and normal.

Malinowski by implication assailed Lévy-Bruhl's theory

that in the primitive the boundaries of the self are not clearly defined and that individuality is almost completely submerged in solidarity with the group. In discussing the factors of social cohesion in the primitive tribes of the Trobriand Islands he demonstrates that the contention of clan-unity is only partly true. Those who have insisted upon clan-unity have tended to be duped by mistaking a legal idea for the sociological realities of tribal life. At certain times, especially in the ceremonial phases of native life, clan-unity does dominate everything, but in general the clan is homogeneous only with regard to other clans. Within the clan or sub-clan there is a strict watch over particular self-interest; a thoroughly business-like spirit prevails and it is not devoid of suspicion, jealousy and mean practices; strained relations between individuals are not infrequent, and strong hatreds, acts of violence and hostility, occur between them. Other anthropologists have advanced like considerations with regard to different primitive communities.

The arguments of Bartlett and Malinowski have very considerable weight. Nevertheless one cannot set aside completely the evidence marshalled by Lévy-Bruhl. One must avoid sharp, artificial antitheses and the pressing of speculations too far beyond ascertained facts. One must recognize that practices and beliefs realistically determined and those determined by phantasy or emotion co-exist in all communities and all individuals, but that the relative emphasis varies. It does seem to be true that the modes of thinking, named "pre-logical" by Lévy-Bruhl, are commoner in primitive than in advanced communities. One might here note the point long ago made by G. F. Stout that since conceptual thinking chiefly depends on language as a tool, the differences between the syntactical usage of the flexional Indo-Germanic languages and of those languages which employ such devices as syncretism and incapsulation necessarily imply differences in mode of thinking. These differences tend to be obliterated by the spread of West-European culture to communities not speaking an Indo-Germanic language, but they remain in full force in the more primitive communities. It also seems to be true that the feeling of individuality is more sharply defined in modern industrial civilization than among primitives, though it is far from absent among them.

Returning again to the resemblance between schizophrenic thinking and that ascribed to pre-literate man, one should note the point that well attested cases of schizophrenia have been found in several primitive societies—Asiatic, American–Indian, Eskimo and Polynesian. This speaks strongly against any simple identification of schizophrenic thought processes with those normal in a non-technical or pre-literate community. Whatever may be the truth in the controversial matter of primitive thinking, it is the case that schizophrenic behaviour often closely corresponds to the modes of thought ascribed by Lévy-Bruhl and the Freudian anthropologists to the uncivilized. Transductive reasoning, notions of duality or bipresence of the individual, ambivalence of feeling, magical practices and ideas, rituals, beliefs of an animistic nature, can frequently be demonstrated in clinical examination or by special tests. The parallel of schizophrenic to primitive beliefs is sometimes extraordinarily close, as I shall show later in a special instance. One must, however, take great care in establishing that such beliefs are not current in the *milieu* from which the patient derives and are therefore unrelated to his illness. One must also remember that there is no sharp contrast between primitive and advanced communities in the matters of magic, animism and related phenomena: there is merely a gradation in their incidence and in the emphasis laid upon them, from pre-technological societies through agricultural communities down to the communities of modern industrialism. The apparent return of the schizophrenic to ways of thinking more magical and animistic than those current in our society is best regarded as a weakening in his conceptual or categorical thinking so that it approximates to the level of conceptual or categorical thinking standard in the pre-literate communities,

About the causes of schizophrenia there are many hypotheses. No single one is sufficient to account for all the factors of so complex and many-sided a phenomenon; most of the explanations put forward are only part of the truth. It is not my intention to add to their number. I wish rather to start from the most comprehensive generalization possible about the symptomatology of schizophrenia; to relate this to facts from certain other biological fields—neurological, psychological, psycho-pathological and pharmacological; and to see what light can be thrown in this way on the phenomenon of schizophrenic painting and its motivation. Such a generalization can be found in Magnan's description of schizophrenia. He states that in schizophrenia a noxious agent erodes the personality and that the demarcation between ego and non-ego begins to disappear, and is finally dissolved as the disease progresses. This generalization subsumes many, though not all, of the symptoms of schizophrenia described at the beginning of the chapter; it would be difficult to find any generalization subsuming more of the symptoms, except the bare statement that they are all of queer or eccentric behaviour. Magnan's generalization describes, and does no more than describe. It does not imply that the noxious agent is either physiogenic or psychogenic in kind. The nature of "ego" and "non-ego" is left unspecified, but "ego" can be taken to denote something having clearly marked boundaries in spatial and temporal reality. If the "ego" boundaries are eroded, the "ego" is no longer distinct from its spatial and temporal surroundings; reality for the ego is changed. Under such conditions thinking, which is a functional relation between the ego and the non-ego, can hardly remain realistic.

The concept "ego", however, is exceedingly unsatisfactory; furthermore, the use of "ego" leads to a biological impasse. It denotes something imaginary like the mathematical point. To substitute "body" for the construct "ego" provides a suitable operational term, capable of biological treatment; it can be observed and verified. As Sherrington emphasized, the "I" is aware of itself as an embodied "I", but the feeling of "I" or "self" is usually wider than the body, sometimes narrower, more rarely co-extensive with it, but through all transformations of this feeling the body remains as the one constant factor. The feeling is wider when "self" is extended to include clothes, implements such as a pen or weapons such as a gun, vehicles such as a bicycle, dependents and subordinates, or friends and comrades; it will be noted that the ease and security with which these can be included in the "ego" vary in degree. The feeling of "self" becomes narrower than the body when the individual is engaged in thinking or intellectual activity or appraisement of his own deeds and qualities; this retraction of the self would appear to be uncommon except in the highly intelligent or intellectually sophisticated. The feeling of "self" may perhaps become co-extensive with the body when the individual is lying in a hot bath. All such statements rest solely on introspective evidence in a matter where introspection is extremely difficult; there are great individual differences. Certain psychologists have attempted by introspection to localize the feeling of "self" in the body. E. Claparede placed it between the two eyes; others have placed it in the thorax. Here, too, individual differences come into play. Moreover, much depends on the activity in which the organism is engaged. The feeling of "self" may well be located between the two eyes when the individual is busied upon an intellectual activity with the body relatively passive—for example, playing chess or reading a book. If the whole body is in motion as in swimming or playing tennis, the feeling of "self" could hardly be located in so limited a spot. It will now be quite plain that this shifting point (or region) whose locality rests on such tenuous and variable introspective evidence is something quite unsuitable for objective scientific treatment. Instead one must make use of the constant component, the verifiable and observable fact; that is, the body itself.

I am now led to the neuro-physiological concept of the "body-image". This phenomenon was first demonstrated by Sir Henry Head on the basis of his work with brain-

injured patients. From studying certain effects of lesions
of the brain—impairment in voluntary movement, impairment in knowledge of the spatial position of the limbs,
loss of touch-localization—Head concluded that the
human organism has two "models" or "schemata" of
itself, the postural model based on kinaesthetic sensation
and the surface model based on cutaneous sensation.
These two models are closely interconnected but the
surface one is the less transient. The postural model is
always being built up and constantly changing by means
of perpetual alterations in position. Head also distinguished the "schema-building" which is an activity in
progress from the "schema-built" which is a state resulting from the activity. Other neurologists have added to
these propositions and modified them. Lhermitte emphasized that vestibular and particularly visual sensations
together with the kinaesthetic and tactile ones were the ·
raw material of a synthesis which constituted the "body-
image". Pötzl, Gerstmann and others, by observing
patients with vascular catastrophes of the temporo-
parietal part of the cerebral cortex, demonstrated that the
nervous integration of the "body-image" lies in that
region. Unawareness of parts of the body occurs without
loss of sensation (anaesthesia); these investigators took
this fact as demonstrating that the disturbance in the
"body-image" is not sensory in nature but is a specific
symptomatology due to a lesion of a specific area. Those
findings about the localization of the "body-image" were
also supported by Hoff's experiments; he was able by
freezing the temporo-parietal region through a skull-
defect to demonstrate unawareness of the opposite body
side (autotopagnosia). Bychowsky stated that the "body-
image" alters not only with body movements and body
positions but also through acquired skill. Neurologists
classify the "body-image" disturbances as positive and
negative. Positive disturbances occur when a patient
apprehends as still present a part of the body that has
been removed. The chief phenomenon here is that of
"phantom-limbs", exhaustively studied by Head and G.

Riddoch; when a limb is amputated the patient has for a long time a sensation that it is still there. Allied to this is the more general phenomenon called anosognosia, or rejection of the evidence of bodily disease. Thus the patient with hemiplegia or paralysis on one side of the body may deny that he is paralysed, the blind man may deny his loss of vision, and so on. Negative disturbances occur when the patient apprehends part of his body as not belonging to him. When the patient suffering in this way is shown an arm he may deny that it belongs to him. Disturbances of this kind occur after lesions of the temporo-parietal region and refer to the opposite side of the body. Purden Martin raises the question, "What would happen if following an extensive bilateral lesion a patient lost the awareness of both halves of his body?" He goes on that the patient "would then be to himself a disembodied spirit. Can you imagine yourself without any body-consciousness? To yourself you could be a disembodied spirit, entirely devoid of body. I find that I am quite unable to imagine myself as such. I can imagine myself possessed of a body of which I was unaware of bodily sensation, and then I would, I suppose, if I remained conscious at all, still be aware of my environment—through eyes and ears of which I was unaware—and I might see my body as I see that of another person. But could I remain conscious if I had no awareness of my body as me? Certainly a large part of consciousness would be lost". Lesions of the left parietal region in right-handed persons occasion finger agnosia, an inability to select and recognize the fingers of either the patient's own hand or of the examining physician's; this is associated with loss of ability to write, to calculate sums and to discriminate between right and left. The foregoing account sketches very briefly the main findings of pure neurology upon awareness of the body and its parts, their existence, spatial position and relations.

The neurological findings clearly raise a number of psychological considerations to which I must now turn. The psychologists of two generations ago, in England notably James Ward and G. F. Stout, devoted some attention to awareness of the body, to the way in which it was singled out as a separate thing from the environment, to its importance as the spatial centre from which the position, distance and direction of other perceived objects are reckoned, and so on. Since that time, however, the whole subject has been largely disregarded in theoretical psychology. The main development and elaboration of psychology in relation to the "body-image" can be found in a series of brilliant studies by the neuro-psychiatrist P. Schilder and his co-workers. He concluded that the "body-image" is a configuration or "Gestalt". He investigated the building up of the "body-image" in children and noted the importance of socialization or identification with others in this regard. He studied the rôle of mirrors in connection with the body-image; he also studied "body-image" experiences in dancing and when travelling in lifts or aeroplanes. He noted that the "body-image" extends in space and implies space perception; he studied its time-relations. He was the first to raise the problem of the perception of internal body-parts, and of feelings of heaviness and lightness. He advanced a theory that primitive space-perception originates in connection with the body openings, the mouth, the anus and the others. His co-worker, L. Bender, affirmed that the occurrence of phantom limbs was a configurational activity. Schilder's view that the "body-image" is a "Gestalt" led to the proposition, obvious enough and yet ignored by the purely neurological investigators, that what goes on in the body is always part of a total situation in which the outer world as well as the body itself is involved.

Fundamental and seemingly exhaustive as the work of Schilder is, much in it is yet obscure and confused. His experimental findings are never presented in an explicit and verifiable form. He depended largely on introspective data with all the pitfalls that such dependence implies. He ignored the relevance of individual differences and seems to have applied inadequate control or systematic variation of conditions. If, however, the criticism in the following paragraph appears to reflect mainly on his work, it is because he opened up paths which others have not ventured to tread.

It must first be noted that though the term "body-image" is now well established, it is a very unfortunate one and Head's original term "body schema" would have been much more appropriate. Except in relation to optics and the theory of vision the term "image" has for many decades in psychology had one meaning only, that is, an experience which reproduces or copies in part with some degree of sensory realism a previous perceptual experience in the absence of the original sensory stimulation. Alternatively it is an element of experience which is centrally aroused and which possesses all the attributes of sensation. These definitions might be taken to apply to the phenomenon of the phantom limb; they certainly do not apply to most of the phenomena comprised in the term "body-image". The chief psychological categories involved in this matter are not images but percepts and concepts.

A second and more important criticism of the term "body-image", advanced by Mr. J. P. S. Robertson, is—and I agree—that in the discussion of Schilder and others it is used to denote a number of quite distinct though connected psychological phenomena. It is often not clear which of these is meant; arguments and demonstrations appropriate to one are quite unwarrantably transferred to another. A clear distinction of these phenomena is of the utmost importance in discussing schizophrenic symptomatology and schizophrenic painting. They are the following:

I. The total complex of sensations or percepts from the body and concerning it at a given moment. Any or all of the sense-modalities may be involved. In the waking organism sensations of touch and proprioceptive and vestibular sensations are always involved; and also sensations of sight, except when the organism is awake with eyes closed. Sensations of hearing are included if the organism is itself uttering sounds and in various other circumstances. Interoceptive sensations of heat and cold and pain are often concerned. In special though rare circumstances even sensations of smell and taste may be included. This complex, if one likes, may be called a configuration. It is in continual change and the emphasis falls now on one sense-modality, now on the other.

II. The individual's feeling of "me, here, now". This depends in part on the sensation-complex just described; it can be shaken seriously or otherwise by disturbances in that complex or contradictory testimony from different modalities. It also depends on factors independent of the sensation-complex; memory, perception and knowledge of the immediate environment; and awareness of the immediate goals toward which the organism is striving.

III. The individual's relatively permanent and static concept or schema of his own body and its parts, their spatial relations and proportions, their qualities, their abilities, disabilities and inabilities. Changes in the sensation-complex can affect this concept only in exceptional or pathological circumstances. The schema has a number of aspects and emphases which differ from time to time and individual to individual, but for the most part it remains clearly defined and static for each normal individual from the end of the period of physical growth. It changes slowly in response to the changes of senescence, perhaps lagging behind them. In special circumstances, particularly with the maimed, disabled and handicapped, there may be two such concepts, one realistic and one idealized, closely similar but differing in the presence or absence of the disability.

IV. The individual's concept or schema of the human body in general, that is, the bodies of other people, their spatial proportions, qualities and so on. This is particularly brought to light in drawings. The concept seems to be completely formed by the end of the period of physical growth, if not somewhat before. It is even more permanent and static than the individual's concept of his own body and is realistic except

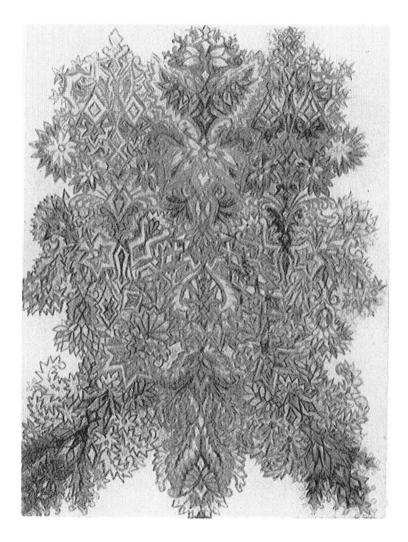

Fig. 7. Cat

face p. 54

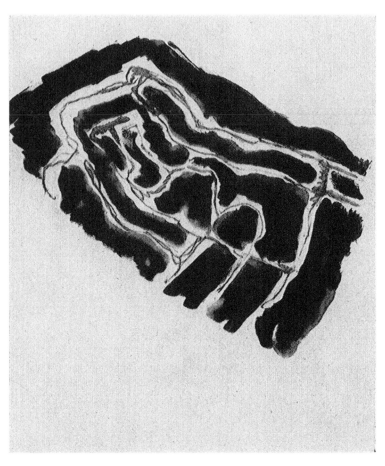

Fig. 8. Painting Under Mescalin

in pathological cases. There is, of course, a separate though similar schema for each sex. This concept seems to be less detailed than the individual's concept of his own body and for the most part it is based on visual sensation alone. It has not received as much attention from other investigators as it deserves.

One must here point out that in the everyday goal-seeking activities of the normal individual these four phenomena are always in the background of the organism's effort, never in the centre. They come to the front only when there is a dysfunction in some part (or the whole), mild or serious, or when the individual for some reason or other adopts a special introspective attitude.

To show the importance of distinguishing the phenomena just enumerated, one may first refer to one of Schilder's investigations. In considering "body-image' experiences when going up or down in lifts he noted that the body in stopping after going down tends to be telescoped and in stopping after ascending, elongated; the feet vary in relation to the head; there are differences in the feelings of lightness or heaviness. One can call these changes in the "body-image" if one likes. They are certainly changes in the sensation-complex of the given moment; they are unlikely to affect the individual's feeling of identity and still less likely to affect his concept of his own body. While such changes can be discriminated by the careful introspective observer they are completely disregarded by the millions who go up and down in lifts every day, busy about their immediate goals; they have no effect, it is all but certain, on the concept those people hold about their own bodies, any more than the optical phenomena discriminated by the careful introspectionist affect the visual perception of his environment.

It should be noted that the sensation-complex, the schema of the individual's own body and the schema of the human body in general, may all refer to the body as a whole or to any of its principal parts. A special rôle in regard to body-parts in the body-schemata is played by the sex organs, because, as many writers have noted, the social ban on their mention or exposure co-exists with a strong interest in them. One must observe the importance of the fact without discussing the many theories of the cause of the ban.

Light on the various "body-image" phenomena is thrown by the cases of deaf-blind individuals such as Helen Keller. Her account of the way in which she apprehends the bodies of others and the human body in general makes it quite clear that her concept is very different from that of persons with an intact sensorium. Her concept is one built upon kinaesthetic data and data of touch, of the sensation of heat and cold, and of smell. She has related this as nearly as she can to the terms in which the normal apprehension of the bodies of others is described, but the final product is something quite different. Her schema of her own body too, it would appear, with its absence of the components of sight and hearing, differs basically from the schema which normal individuals have of their own bodies.

Distinguishing the four "body-image" phenomena I have enumerated is important chiefly in relation to schizophrenia, as I have already indicated. In cases of demonstrable organic lesion, it is the changes in the perceptual complex which are mainly emphasized; the changes in the body concept are not so prominent. Moreover, the emphasis lies on changes in parts of the body and not the body as a whole. A special manifestation of schizophrenic "body-image" disturbance should be noted at this point; schizophrenic patients are frequently observed to pinch themselves in the face or elsewhere to assure themselves that they really are there, as substantial beings. In schizophrenic symptomatology, however, while there may be quite often a disturbance of the feeling of identity, of the concepts of the individual's own body, and of the concept of the human body in general, a disturbance in the sensation-complex is less readily demonstrable. But that such a disturbance is likely to exist is suggested by certain psycho-physiological experiments, using a pharmacological technique which I am about to describe.

Before doing so I wish to summarize the ground we have covered so far: schizophrenic symptoms may be characterized in the most general way by saying that the boundaries of the ego are eroded by a noxious agent; the ego is for empirical treatment equated to the body or rather the "body-image"; this concept includes three phenomena which frequently show manifest disturbance in schizophrenia; these three phenomena are distinct from but dependent on a fourth phenomenon which does not show manifest disturbance in schizophrenia; it will be demonstrated now that disturbances artificially induced in this fourth phenomenon can lead to disturbance in the other three.

In relating schizophrenic symptomatology to "body-image" disturbance some aspects may seem excluded. The motor-symptoms, mannerisms and postures would appear to have a fairly close relation, at any rate for the most part. The loss of affect, the somatic delusions, the feelings of depersonalization, have an obvious close connection. Certain of the other thinking disorders may seem less obviously included. Here a brief account of the building up of the "body-image" in the child is appropriate. The child builds up its concept of itself on the basis of the sensory data already noted as constituting the body sensation-complex; these are conjoined with ceaseless motor activity and experimentation. The child's own name becomes a fixating point. A continual process of comparison of itself with other selves reinforces the child's concept of itself and builds up its concept of the human body in general. The segregation of its own body from the spatial environment is usually accomplished before the second year, according to Koffka; knowledge of spatial and temporal relations is built up slowly but nearly reaches maturity by about the tenth year, as noted by Sturt and others. A distinction between the animate and inanimate environment is learnt securely only in late childhood; it is easily lost in the adult. This is important in relation to acquiring the knowledge that thoughts and feelings can be private to oneself. There seems to be no

satisfactory evidence of when children learn that their
thoughts cannot be read, but can at the most be guessed;
but accounts of the study of lies at different ages suggest
that the knowledge comes late in childhood. The notion
that feelings are not private persists beyond childhood
and is never entirely lost by the adult; the ready com-
municability of feeling to the human environment gives it
some semblance of truth. Most adults are at times guilty
of Ruskin's "pathetic fallacy", that the inanimate environment, the plants and the animals, participate in our
feelings of the moment. The notion is stronger in childhood. All this suggests that the weakness of the boundaries
of the self in the schizophrenic, shown in ideas of reference
and influence, and in other symptoms, may plausibly be
treated as a weakening of the "body-image" so that its
contours are no stronger than in early childhood; "body-
image" can here be taken to denote both the feeling of
identity, "me-here-now", and the concept of the body.
To state this is not necessarily to imply a regressive theory
of schizophrenia.

Evidence on the effect of disturbance in the sensation
complex upon the feeling of identity, the individual body-
concept, and the general concept of others' bodies will
now be offered. It has to do chiefly with the use of mescalin
once more. Mescalin was employed by Guttmann on
60 normal subjects in order to induce what could be regarded as an experimental psychosis. Producing as it does
an introspective and hallucinatory state, mescalin intoxication most characteristically results in altered visual perception, in "body-image" disturbances, and in disturbed
spatial and temporal experiences. The visual hallucinations are of both a simple and a composite kind. The
hallucinatory pictures change constantly and fluctuate;
and they have been clearly described by one of Guttmann's subjects, who said, "When I happened to look at
a burning cigarette it started sparkling like fireworks; the
whole room was filled with small fiery stars. If the cigarette
was moved, circles, oblongs and other shapes appeared".
Other subjects reported that perception of their own

bodies became altered; they noticed that their limbs changed size and shape independently of visual perception and uninfluenced by it. One said that he had a numb feeling of the mouth as if there were a swelling of his lips; "the skin was unusually vivid". Another said, "I lost control of the position of my face . . . I pulled faces."

Alterations in experiences of space and time may be illustrated by further statements. One subject had a feeling that his body was inseparable from the surrounding space: another reported that gradually the feeling of body vanished and the position of the limbs could not be localized: "The posture of the body could hardly be determined, it could scarcely be separated from its surroundings." Space for these subjects had new dimensions, new qualities. Time also became altered. One subject reports: "I drank a spoonful of soup and looked around me and looked down again at my plate. It had been in front of me for hundreds of years, but my movements and conversation at the table were no slower than in ordinary life; indeed they appeared somewhat accelerated. I must have kept everyone waiting." The breakdown of the boundaries between the self and the environment is also well described by the subject who said, "all demarcation melts away; one feels lost in the cosmos". Derealization is illustrated by the observation that "all doings and sayings of the people around me were absolutely unintelligible to me, like the rules of a strange game". A disturbance of conceptual thinking was experienced in some mescalin-intoxicated subjects in a direct and simple form. One reported: "Each word I thought was connected with a picture. This hindered me thinking, as the concrete picture held me."

Such experiences have been reproduced by other experimenters with mescalin. Hashish and marihuana have been used to produce experiences of a similar nature. This strongly suggests that the noxious agent in schizophrenia first operates on the complex of body sensations and from there affects the other "body-image" phenomena.

Several other features of the mescalin experiments are of importance, namely:

I. The disturbed perception of space and time. It will have been evident at many points in the account of the "body-image" phenomena, especially the "me-here-now" feeling, that they depend upon a clear perception of space and time. These experiments lead one to believe that adequate perception of space and time depends also upon an unimpaired complex of body sensations.

II. The impairment of ordered conceptual thinking: verbal symbols were replaced by visual images.

III. The fact that the visual hallucinations might be regarded as creative experiences of an unusually intense kind.

These last two features make it necessary to set out some views upon "visualistic" thinking. In early childhood, thinking tends to be in terms mainly of visual images. For the child there are, to begin with, no true symbols but only imaginal representations of meaning. Gradually the child learns to think in terms of verbal symbols devoid of intrinsic meaning. The visual symbols themselves tend to be altered in quality as the child grows older, so that they become schematic or conceptual. A process of condensation and stylization takes place, which is analogous in a certain degree to the development of hieroglyphics from picture-writing. According to Goldstein and his followers the development of pictorial part-images into abstract concepts is one which is not complete until the onset of puberty, and which shows parallelism to the development of the ego. Most psychologists would regard this as rather over-simplified and lacking in experimental demonstration; in some children visualistic thinking disappears long before puberty; on the other hand, some adults show it in a marked degree. Apparently, however, the more concretistic elements of thinking tend to disappear at puberty. Visualistic thinking is clearly related to the eidetic imagery found by Jaensch to be prevalent in children and to disappear, save in a minority of cases, at puberty. Jaensch postulated three genetic levels or stages of imagery—the after-sensation, the eidetic image and finally the true memory image which is the basis of conceptual thinking. This suggests that visual imagery fades with the development of conceptional thinking. Conversely perhaps alterations in conceptual thinking due to pathology may show a return to predominantly visualistic thinking.

An interesting contribution of electro-physiology to eidetic studies and mescalin intoxication is worth considering. Electro-encephalographic records show alteration in the resting alpha rhythm of the visual cortex when the eidetic subject experiences eidetic images. Chweitzer and his colleagues found that the onset of the effect of the mescalin flattens the alpha rhythm; this flattening coincides with altered time-space perception and with the onset of visual hallucinations. These findings underline the markedly physiological character of what in psychological terms was called "visualistic" thinking.

In schizophrenics it would appear that some concepts disintegrate into pictorial part-images again as if under the influence of mescalin; there is an increased emphasis on the perceptual as opposed to the conceptual elements in thinking. It seems reasonable to believe also that in primitives there is a similar emphasis on the perceptual, though in the absence of empirical evidence one hesitates to affirm it. This disintegration of concepts appears to be accompanied by a weakening of conceptual time and space relation (possibly of perceptual time and space experiences as well), of the feeling of identity and of the schemata of the individual's own body and of the bodies of others. Possibly all these phenomena depend on alteration in the complex of body-sensations. At any rate, reality is altered for the schizophrenic. The weakening in his conceptual and categorical mode of thought brings it about that for the most part he does not think realistically but in a way that appears magical or animistic. Perhaps it would be truer to the facts to say that realistic thinking

becomes relatively weakened and non-categorical thinking, giving an appearance of magic or animism, relatively
strengthened. The increased tendency to non-categorical
thinking is itself dependent on body-image disturbance,
loss of boundaries between the body and its outer environment, and distorted time-space relations.

Schizophrenic paintings can now be presented as active
rituals of a creative sort. They are outcomes of a mode of
thinking that is predominantly non-categorical. The
schizophrenic paints to adjust himself to his altered
reality. He recreates the world so that it shall harmonize
with his experience. He has no message about the real
world, directed to its inhabitants; he is trying to express
an altered world. Not only have his concepts broken up
into pictorial fragments; his total personality has done so
too. The content of his pictures is determined by his
thought disturbances. The fragmentation of the personality directly depends on the disordered "body-image",
the disordering of the concept of his own body and of the
bodies of others. This is depicted in amputated limbs,
mutilated bodies, detached heads, fusion of parts and the
like. The weakening in the concept of space-relations (and
possibly in their perception) is revealed in a poor presenta-
tion of perspective and a general lack of spatial unity—
the picture is not clearly defined and set off from the
space surrounding it. The disturbance in conceptual (and
perhaps perceptual) time is shown in the depiction of
successive temporal events as simultaneous, and in allied
phenomena; this resembles what we see, for example, in
pre-renaissance painting but, whereas in the latter it depends on a difference of aim and an absence of knowledge
which was to be acquired later (a lack of skill), in the
schizophrenic it is primarily dependent on disorder of
thinking. It would be naïve, however, to expect to find
each single symptom neatly expressed in schizophrenic
pictures. They are a general representation of the patient's
disturbed thinking. They often have a peculiar appeal
through their mixture of drawing with "writing in", that
is, naming what is drawn. This may be regarded as a

mixture of elements primarily conceptual (writing) with elements primarily perceptual (drawing).

The previous chapter and the present one have both tended to show that in all human activity, normal or abnormal, the psychological and the physiological are closely intermingled. Psychotic art should be evaluated as an expression of such psycho-physiological unity. Perception is inseparable from motivity, as demonstrated in "body-image" formation by Schilder and elsewhere by others; no strict delineation can be drawn between reception of stimuli and expression. This proposition must be applied to the art products of the psychotic. A purely psychological description is insufficient; they must be appraised physiologically as well. It is not enough to treat them only as reactions in the form of expressive phenomena; nor is it enough to treat them only as receptive reflexions of a new experience of the world. Schizophrenic art contains both expressive and receptive, both motor and sensory, phenomena. These are essentially biological because they can be considered not only in terms of psychology but also in those of physiology.

The advantage of taking an aspect of psychotic art which can be formulated in biological terms is that it more easily allows for experimental research both into the nature of psychosis and into the nature of art either by means of psycho-physiological investigation as in the mescalin experiments or by means (which we shall come to) of psychometric studies. This is the scientific justification of such a method.

IV

AN ILLUSTRATIVE CASE OF
SCHIZOPHRENIA

I

I SHALL NOW illustrate the theoretical conclusions of the previous chapter by means of the case of a 55-year-old labourer suffering from chronic schizophrenia.

Mr. A. was admitted 14 years ago to a psychiatric institution. He then was solitary, self-absorbed, reluctant to answer questions, or to enter into any conversation. He thought that he was "done in" many years ago, and that if he went home he would be killed. Later his delusions became more bizarre; he believed that he was in the secret service, that he understood all the languages of the world. His periods of quiet solitariness alternated with periods of slight excitement. The diagnosis established was schizophrenia. There was no physical abnormality detectable except in his right arm and hand; this arm had been injured in the 1914–1918 war. The power of the right hand was diminished; abduction of the thumb was lost and the thenar eminence was flattened. There was some diminution in sensation over the radial part of his hand. (The physical findings are identical to-day.) He settled down ultimately and partook in the regulated life of a psychiatric institution. A short while ago, however, it was discovered that he made a fair number of rather interesting drawings, which he used to hide from the medical and nursing staff. The case was re-investigated, and I give a summary of these investigations.

The previous history, secured by the Psychiatric Social Worker, has been pieced together from information given by his wife, two of his sisters and three elderly inhabitants of his birthplace, one of whom taught him in the infant school.

Until he was mobilized in 1914, Mr. A. lived in N., a village a few miles from Maidstone and about one mile from a railway station. The family consisted of his father, who was a foreman bricklayer, his mother, two brothers, three sisters and himself; their standard of living was not above, and may have been somewhat below, that of the village in general. His father, now dead, drank to excess, and the home possibly was not a particularly satisfactory one; nevertheless, the father and one of the brothers were steady workers who kept their jobs for a lifetime. The sisters, who entered domestic service at 14, later married and are now leading settled, reasonably comfortable lives. The third brother, said to have been the one with whom Mr. A. was most friendly, is popularly, though not officially, believed to have committed suicide at the age of 27; he was burnt to death in somewhat mysterious circumstances on the eve of his wedding. The mother never recovered from the shock and died within a year, following a breakdown that caused her to be sent to a home.

At school none of the A. family did very well, and Mr. A. was remarkable only for his cruelty to other children when he was himself quite young, and for his interest in drawing. He was quite often in trouble, and was not regarded as one of the "nice boys" of the village, but he mixed with other children and was not considered by himself, his family or the villagers to be outstandingly different from others.

Mr. A.'s work-record differs markedly from that of his father and surviving brother; he began by being apprenticed under his father as a bricklayer, but he never completed the apprenticeship. Instead he made an abortive attempt to join the Army; on his return home he learned hedge-cutting and fencing. Later he set up on his own account in this trade, with six men under him and his wife dealing with the paper work. Before this there had been his army service from 1914 to 1918, an attempt at running his own fried-fish business, and a spell, it seems, of helping with a travelling show.

Mr. A.'s capacity for forming social relationships seems to have diminished as he grew older; as a young man he had no particular friend of his own sex, and he came to mix more and more exclusively with show-people, until after his marriage to one of them he neither had nor wanted any company other than his wife and her family. (He had previously been courting a respectable young domestic servant.) His own family were outraged by his marrying a woman who had no settled home (to make it worse she was a widow with a small daughter) and by his leading a kind of semi-nomadic existence. After his marriage, he had little contact with his family, although his mother became at least partly reconciled to his wife. His last two visits to his old home were made after the deaths of his brother and of his mother. He was greatly distressed at the brother's fate, and was the only one of the family to see his very badly burned remains.

Mr. A. became the father of four sons. One died a few years after Mr. A. was admitted to hospital. Of the others the eldest is married and working on a farm, the second is in the army, and the youngest lives with Mrs. A. and the step-daughter, spending the summer picking fruit in rural Kent and the winter in chopping wood and similar occupations.

The village offered nothing in the way of cultural pursuits and Mr. A.'s interests were very limited. Before his marriage he worked enthusiastically at the family allotment, but he did no gardening afterwards. He was not religious and never went to church after he grew up; he was married in a registry office. He was not concerned with magic or the supernatural, except that at one time he learnt water-divining from the old man who taught him hedge-cutting. He did not show any body-preoccupation and he was right-handed. He never read, nor did he belong to any kind of club or association. He always maintained his liking for drawing apparently, but unfortunately none of his early drawings are now available.

As was mentioned, the neurological condition of his right hand has not changed since the original examination. His general physical health is satisfactory and his appearance is that of a well-nourished elderly man.

The psychiatric and psychometric investigations were conducted simultaneously for reasons which will be self-evident in the description below. The psychological investigations were conducted in a masterly fashion by Mr. J. P. S. Robertson.

The standard tests applied to Mr. A. were the Wechsler-Bellevue Intelligence Scale, the Rorschach Ink-Blot Test, the Thematic Apperception Test, the Group Word-Association Test, the Visual-Motor Gestalt Test and the Pin-Man Test. The Wechsler-Bellevue Scale is a well-known American system of tests for the assessment of adult intelligence, now widely employed in this country as well. The Rorschach and Thematic Apperception Tests are likewise well-known and extensively used in psychological practice; in the first of these the form-perception and phantasies of the patient are examined by showing him a series of ink-blots and asking him to say what they look like or can represent; in the second the patient's phantasies are investigated by showing him a number of pictures depicting ambiguous human situations and asking him to tell a story about each of them. The other three standard tests are less well-known. The Group Word-Association Test has been much used during the last few years in the selection of personnel and is now being applied also in abnormal psychology; the patient in company with others is shown a series of words on cards and asked to write down what each word brings to his mind, a time-limit of fifteen or thirty seconds being imposed. The Visual-Motor Gestalt Test has been developed by L. Bender from the Gestalt Figures of Wertheimer; the patient is shown these figures drawn on small cards and asked either to copy them or to reproduce them from memory; the test discloses various pathological phenomena, especially disturbance in apprehending configurations and in the perception of size. The Pin-Man Test was devised by Reitman and standardized by Robertson; the patient is shown a number of schematized drawings strongly suggesting the expression of different emotional states and is asked to say what feelings they represent or show; the test reveals disturbances in abstract thinking, especially in the conceptualization of emotion, and disorders of body-imagery.

An indication of Mr. A.'s performance on the standard tests will be given in this account. In general his performance in the Wechsler, the Rorschach, the Word-Association and the Pin-Man Test was typically that of a deteriorated schizophrenic; Thematic Apperception was beyond his capacity.

Besides being subjected to the six standard tests Mr. A. was examined to discover how he would judge length of lines, size of squares and circles and duration of empty and filled intervals. The psycho-physical methods of production and single stimuli were used. His memory for the time-order of events was tested in a similar way. The occurrence in him of space and time disturbances suggested the desirability of these investigations. It was apparent, however, that whether or not those disturbances had a perceptual component they were mainly conceptual in character. So special questionnaires had to be designed to elicit his general notions of space, time, cosmology, causality and body-structure and parts. In addition to this an attempt was made to get him to produce drawings under standard conditions.

First of all we must describe his intellectual and educational status, as disclosed by the tests and other examinations. On the Wechsler-Bellevue Scale he rated an intelligence quotient of seventy-eight; that is the level of a border-line mental defective. It is possible by means of this test-scale to estimate the original intelligence-level of demented patients and the extent to which they have deteriorated intellectually. The suggestion here was that Mr. A. was originally of dull normal intelligence, not a mental defective, and that he now shows a pathological degree of intellectual deterioration. In this test-scale his efficiency of performance fluctuated from one sub-test to the other in a manner characteristic of schizophrenics. His educational status is low. He reads laboriously, having much trouble over comparatively simple words; most words longer than a monosyllable he spells out letter by letter; he cannot read to himself silently but articulates each word aloud. His spelling is approximate and marked by frequent omissions of letters and whole syllables. So far as arithmetic is concerned he can carry out sums on the four rules and money calculations with creditable speed and accuracy, but beyond that he can do nothing. He left school at thirteen and a half; his attendance had been somewhat irregular. Taken as a whole, his educational attainment is more or less what would be expected in a person of his background and history. In discussing the oddity of some of his notions one must at all times bear in mind the extent to which sane individuals of similar intelligence, background and education would express beliefs equally at variance with modern knowledge.

Throughout the tests modes of behaviour recurred again and again and certain beliefs were repeatedly stated. The first general feature of his behaviour was that he was almost completely unable to consider any question except in direct relation to himself and his past experiences. He could view nothing in a detached manner. The dull and the ignorant not infrequently show this characteristic in a mild form but as will shortly be evident in Mr. A. the tendency becomes extreme. To the question in the Wechsler test: "Why does the state require people to sign a register when they get married?" his reply was: "I write a form out for them to show they're legally married." To another question: "Why are laws necessary?" he responded: "Because my work has to be paid for." When asked what he would do if he were the first person to discover an outbreak of fire in a cinema, he said, "I don't go to the pictures!" and could not be persuaded to consider the question further. Again, when asked to find something similar about a coat and a dress he replied: "I was always well-dressed. I always used to wear a coat"; and would add nothing more. Three constructed accounts of incidents were read to him, resembling real incidents in his life-history but having also a number of distinguished characteristics; one concerned a bicycle-accident, one a fire and one a chase by a bull. He was able to deal with them only in terms of the true autobiographical occurrence and could not introduce the modifications or incorporate the divergent details required by the constructed story. Such inability to detach the self from a presented situation is noted by Goldstein as a principal manifestation of pathological concreteness of attitude. It is especially characteristic of organic cases but is also frequent in deteriorated schizophrenics.

The same tendency was shown in the Pin-Man Test where he apprehended the figures as pictures of himself in different postures, in the Rorschach where most of the blots bécame objects or incidents in his past history, and in the Thematic Apperception Test so far as he was able to do it.

A somewhat different but allied tendency was his habit of identifying himself with every rôle or function of importance that was mentioned. Thus he claimed at different times to have fulfilled almost every possible occupation. Thus when asked about marriage in the registry office he had replied "I write out a form for them." At another point he claimed to be a doctor: "I know all about diseases and can cure them all. I know what's wrong with everybody." Again he asserted that he was a clergyman: "I can make any child into a priest or a vicar by christening him." At other points he claimed to be a lawyer, a judge, to know all about weaving and textiles, all about explosives and chemicals, all about colours and painting, about building and road-making. When asked, "Who is the present king of England?" he answered, "Well, I'm

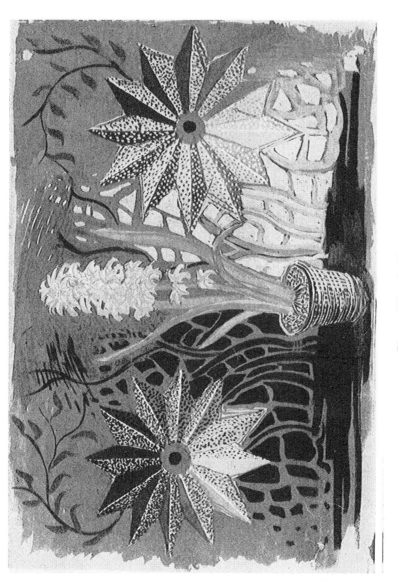

Fig. 9. 'Hyacinth'

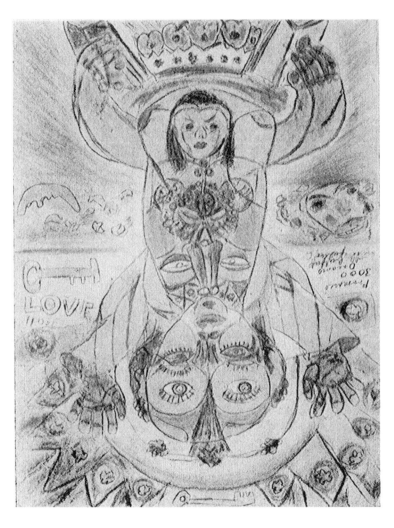

Fig. 10. Doodle

one of them"; when asked, "How long ago did Christ live?" he replied, with apparent astonishment, "He's still alive. I'm Christ and I'm here." The shifting and unstable character of these grandiose notions will be apparent. They were expressed side by side with his more stabilized conception of himself as a farmer, producing food for the whole world, which will shortly be described.

Together with this identification of himself with occupations or offices of importance there ran a continual tendency to compare himself with the examiner, mainly so far as physique or dress was concerned, in a way quite irrelevant to the matter under discussion. Several times he remarked, "Here we are sitting side by side, you sitting there, me sitting here." Once he added to this, "You've got a strong constitution. I got a strong constitution." Another time he added, "Some people have got more hair than others, on their body and all. Me and you are not baldheaded, are we?" On still another occasion he said, "You got your hat off. I take my hat off", suiting the action to the word. He persisted in regarding all the test-material, the Wechsler drawings, the Rorschach Ink Blots, the Thematic Apperception pictures, the Pin-Man figures, as art products of the examiner; he expressed his contempt for them in no unmeasured terms! "That's a useless drawing, that is. Is that all you can do? I can do better than that any day." His main grounds of criticism were that these drawings were not of living people—"They're all dead, all lifeless"—whereas his drawings were drawings of people "with life in 'em, like you and me sitting here. We're alive." He also criticized the Thematic Apperception drawings and a map of the hospital as being "placed" or "hung round" "the wrong way"; it was not possible to clarify what he meant by this.

Another form of identification along apparently distinct lines was the identification of himself with inanimate objects depicted on the cards. In the Wechsler scale there is a picture-completion test in which the patient is shown drawings of objects or situations where something is missing and is required to say what it is. One of these is of a

6

watch where the second hand is absent; the patient looked at it and remarked "There's a dent in its side where an artery has been opened up and is bleeding and the doctor has tried to stop the bleeding with a pebble." Much later in the examination he narrated an incident during the First World War when he had been wounded in the arm, an artery had been ruptured and the army-surgeon, according to his account, had arrested the bleeding with a pebble. Another of these pictures represents a door without a handle; here he answered, "The keyhole is there, but my posterior is missing; there is no human posterior on it." His preoccupation with the posterior we shall come to presently. There were several other less clear examples of identification with inanimate objects.

His verbal behaviour showed some characteristic features. There was an extreme repetition of certain automatic phrases appropriately and inappropriately, especially: "All different answers to that", "I'll prove it to you", and "I proved it to you when I was a baby". He made great use of a neologism, "convertical", of variable and vague meaning but usually denoting some sort of spatial, temporal or causal relation: "The apple-tree was convertical to the glass-house", "The motor-car moves because the petrol is convertical in the engine", "It must be Tuesday because my pension is convertical on Wednesday". He exhibited the phenomenon of associating his thoughts by means of homonyms; this might be considered a form of confusion between words and things. It gives the appearance of paronomasia, but his attitude was not that of someone making a pun. Examples of this are the following: when asked to say what "fur" meant, he said, "Fur is fur because it goes fur" (i.e. far); he described people in the world as "needies" because they "need everything, clothes, food and all what you eat, same as you need plant to make the things, and don't you knead bread?"

Besides the repetition of automatic phrases he showed other forms of perseveration. Notions and words from an answer to one question often intruded with marked inappropriateness into the next answer or the next answer but one. Several times there was a failure to answer a question correctly and then at a later point he offered the right answer to that question but in response to quite a different one. There was also periodically a perseverative return to matters raised by the examiner in the early part of the testing. This was quite distinct from the perseveration of his special pre-occupations. Some of these perseverative phenomena are more commonly seen in organic than schizophrenic cases.

He was not infrequently unable to find words for the meaning he wanted to express and he indicated it by some form of concrete representation. Thus when asked to say what "diamond" meant he could not define it in words but demonstrated the shape by an ingenious interdigitation of his fingers. Similarly he attempted to express the meaning of the word microscope (misconceived as telescope) by a miming representation of someone looking out to sea through a spy-glass. There were a number of such gestural or miming representations. This method of expressing meanings by using gesture or concrete representation in substitution for or supplementation of verbal statement is not at all uncommon in people of Mr. A.'s background and cultural status. Nevertheless in his case it appeared to go beyond the usual and to reach pathological proportions. Several times in the early stages of the testing he appeared to be in need of paper and pencil to show pictorially what he wanted to say. Accordingly, paper and pencil were placed in front of him to use when he felt it necessary. This technique, however, was not so successful as might be expected. There was extreme difficulty in distracting his attention from a drawing once he had begun on it; once started he would continue a process of painstaking elaboration which impeded the general application of the tests.

Mr. A. exhibited several preoccupations: the most outstanding of these, both by reason of its unusual character and its frequent repetition, was the delusion that he was right outside the world, though apparently spatially in it.

Most people were in the world; in particular the examiner and the hospital authorities were very definitely there; but besides Mr. A. miners and quarrymen and fishermen were also outside the world. The birds of the air were outside the world and so were sea-fish and river-fish. This notion invited further investigation; it raised interesting problems about Mr. A.'s ideas of cosmology and his orientation in conceptual space.

In so strange a situation, apparently in the world and yet in fact outside it, Mr. A. had a very important task to perform. Most usually he described it as that of growing or producing food to maintain all the people in the world. Food, he insisted, came from outside the world. Sometimes he associated "other farmers, all the farmers in the world" with himself in the execution of this task; most usually he presented it as incumbent on himself alone. Other forms that the task assumed were that of "making everybody in the world wise", that of "curing all the diseases in the world", and that of "mending all the roads and repairing all the buildings in the world". These were not treated as parallel activities; each was presented at a given moment as the entire and sole nature of the task. Further aspects of this task will be described in discussing Mr. A.'s notions of cosmology. In order to complete the task he was compelled to live for "twenty hundred years"; he never varied this number, however often he mentioned it. He spoke of the task at all times with great feeling and conviction. All attempts to ascertain who had imposed the task were quite unsuccessful; it was clear, however, that no theological component was involved in the idea.

A second, apparently quite distinct, preoccupation, already referred to, was with body-parts, more precisely with the posterior and the anus. This found expression on a number of occasions though not nearly so frequently or insistently as the preoccupation just described. His remark when identifying himself with a picture of a door on one of the Wechsler cards has already been noted. In doing the Group Word-Association Test his response to the

word "alcohol" was "Kee-hole, a . . . hole" (*sic*) and to
the word "body" it was simply "hole". On the Rorschach
Test he saw in the blots on four separate occasions "the
human posterior" or "organs in the human posterior";
the nature of these "organs" was vague and he could not
specify them—they were neither the bowels nor the sex
organs, he stated. The oddest example of this preoccupation emerged when he was asked which season of the year
it was. He replied, "It's the corn season. I sow all the
corn this month. That's why I got all the land in the
world ready this month. I did it together with all the
farmers in the world. The corn what we put in this month,
I'll prove it to you." Here he unexpectedly turned a most
agile somersault and landed on his hands and feet with
his bottom prominently turned upwards. Supported on
his right hand and toes he pointed with his left hand
repeatedly to his anus and said, "That's the way we do
it. We put it in that way. I'll prove it to you. I proved it
when I was a baby. This is what you do. Farmers and
blacksmiths and all do it." A number of possible explanations of the meaning of this performance will suggest
themselves; he would not elucidate his meaning any
further himself. In particular he denied that he intended
any reference to the manuring of the soil.

The marked disordering in conceptual space and time,
alike evident in his drawings and his curious delusions,
suggested an investigation of his judgments of perceptual
space and time and of his concept of the lengths of short
distances and intervals. Nothing outside normal limits
was revealed here. His verbalized judgments of length of
lines, his production of lines or figures equal in length or
size to a given line or figure, were both accurate to an
extent beyond the average. His reproduction of the
Bender-Gestalt figures was better than the average. His
verbalized judgment of filled and unfilled intervals of
time and his production of intervals equal to a given
interval showed a pronounced tendency to over-estima-
tion, especially in the verbalized judgments; this over-
estimation was considerably greater than is usual, but one

could not say that it was definitely outside normal limits. So far as his memory for time-order was concerned he was tested on his capacity to reproduce a succession of taps on different coloured blocks, some circular and some square. He first began to fail when there was a succession of six taps and he was quite unable to reproduce accurately a succession of more than seven taps. This, however, is a creditable performance for one of his intelligence-level and age.

It will now be of value to describe his general orientation in conceptual space and time. He knew the hour of the day, the day of the week and the month of the year, though he was unable to give any satisfactory ground for his statements. He was out by ten days in stating the day of the month. In explanation of this he said: "I must have missed the days in talking to you." He believed that the year was 1968 and over-estimated his own age by four years. As to the season he could not name it "autumn", but he knew it was the corn season. He was vague about recurring dates such as Armistice Day, Easter and Christmas. He found it easier to regard these in terms of a particular occasion rather than generally; thus when asked in what month Armistice Day falls he replied, "It was in 1918", and in what month Christmas falls he said, "Last Christmas was in December". Later he maintained that there were "two Christmases in the year, one last December and one this". He was sure that the day of the week would be the same in different parts of England. His estimates of how long it would take him to walk or to go by motor-vehicle to different places in the locality or to go by train to places further afield were reasonable. He was able to state his age at leading events in his life, such as leaving school, marriage and the like, with plausible accuracy, though he could not give the year. The only historical events prior to his own life of which he showed any cognizance were the Crimean War and the Indian Mutiny. He could not say when Queen Elizabeth or Napoleon lived. He thought his grandfather would probably have been alive at the same time as Henry VIII.

Such ignorance of historical matters is no more than would be expected in a man so educated and of such origins. More unusual was his insistence that there had been no Second World War: "There ain't been no other war except the one that started in 1914. We know all about that. It's no good keep on saying that. There's only one war and that's outside the world. You can have a million other wars, but only one on the outside of the world." He insisted that a war was going on outside the world, "and all the other wars come in the middle of it", but it was impossible to elucidate any other details about it. When asked how long ago the world began he would only reply: "I go on a-making it." When asked if anything existed before the world began he inquired: "Would there have been fishes and the sea then? That were all, the fishes in the sea." As to the end of the world he observed, "It will never end because I will go on a-making it. I've over twenty hundred years to do on public work."

So far as his orientation in conceptual space was concerned, he was able to describe the relative position of prominent landmarks in the hospital and its grounds with considerable accuracy. He also described accurately the relative positions of sample towns and villages in East Surrey and Kent. He was asked to draw a map of the British Isles; all considered, this was a fair approximation and he was able to point out the position of towns such as London, Canterbury, Manchester and Birmingham with reasonable correctness. There were certain gross errors in the position of the Isle of Man, Ireland and Newhaven (where he had once worked). At a subsequent point he voluntarily corrected all these errors. It should be noted that in referring to the scenes of his earlier life and to the present location of his family he was always curiously vague and spoke of "back there"; it was difficult to make him talk precisely on this matter. About the positions of countries other than the British Isles his knowledge was mixed, in some respects amazingly accurate, in others very inexact. He knew the location of countries in the

Near East very well; he said that he had been there during the 1914–1918 war. He was vague about the position of Russia, "Somewhere near Salonika", and thought that Australia was just beyond Canada and New Zealand just beyond that. Such ignorance of geography is quite in accordance with his educational status; nevertheless it should be remarked that he has at times pored over maps and copied them. These questions were presented by asking to what countries he would come if he flew in an aeroplane north, south, east and west respectively. He denied that it is possible for aeroplanes to fly: "It is all labour in vain," he said, "they fall back to the ground." So the form of the question had to be modified by adding the supposition, "if it were possible to fly", which he accepted. He stated that if anyone went due east or west he would come to the sea and after that there would be nothing but more sea.

Such remarks suggested that Mr. A. did not conceive the world as round. This question was posed to him direct by asking what was the shape of the world. He answered, "It's supposed to be round and I go by the circumference of the world. I believe the world is round meself. All the things you look at is round. Well, the world must be round. You put water into a vessel, well, it's *round* what it holds! There's all different ways with water." It would appear that he knows it to be commonly accepted as a fact that the world is round and that he has seen geographical globes. Nevertheless his own private concept is of a flat earth surrounded by sea. He is in a pit underneath this flat earth "outside the world". Food is underneath the world, that is, "outside it", but comes into it by pushing up as corn and vegetables to feed animal and man. The fish which are in the sea "outside the world" are also brought into it to feed people. His task in his pit or quarry "outside the world" is to force the corn and vegetables to push their way up through the ground. He is similarly able to influence from his pit the catching of the fish. He is also able to affect from his pit "outside the world" the minds of men and to make them wise; he can also affect diseases. This account, of course, renders precise what is in its essence vague and fluid.

With regard to his general cosmology he believes that the sun goes round the earth; he could not at first say what happens to it at night, but afterwords, using a piece of knowledge separate from his private construct of the world, he said it must warm other countries. He stated that the sun, the moon and the stars were all the same distance from the earth and no one knew how far that was. About the sun he observed: "The sun is glory!" He expressed some very interesting notions about the moon: "Each moon gives birth to another moon. The moon wasteth away every month and another one has to grow next month. It's like everybody; it dies and is reborn."

These notions of the world suggested an inquiry into his theological ideas. Already when he had declared, "I am outside the world and all the millions of others are in the world", he had been asked "What about God?" He replied: "That's only a name for a village, that's all that means; Godstone and places like that." When pressed on the point: "Don't you think there is a God, then?" he reiterated: "No, no, that's only a name. That's all named on the map. Godstone is the name of a village." At a later point he answered in similar fashion. He entertains no notions of immortality, apart from his idea that he must live for twenty hundred years. When asked what happens to people after they die, he answered in terms of burial, the graveyard and decay.

In order to elucidate the strong element in his cognitive processes of what some investigators have termed "magical thinking" and others would interpret as "conceptual weakening" he was asked a number of questions about causality. He accounted for the movement of trains, motor-cars, lifts, threshing machines, animals and human beings all in the same manner: "they're started up and once they're started they've just got to go; they keep on going and going." With regard to weather-phenomena, rain, wind, thunder and lightning, he gave an account not meteorologically correct but reasonable for one of his education; thus of lightning he said, "The clouds go together with a bang and that makes lightning." The winds, he said, "come from across the sea outside the world". He rejected most of the common superstitions— the number thirteen, spilling salt, black cats, robins as signs of death and others; but stated, however, that it was bad to walk under ladders. He had already claimed that he could read all the examiner's thoughts and knew in advance every question that he was going to be asked. He now stated that he could read "everybody's thoughts, builders and all". He also stated that he could put thoughts into people's minds because "most people are not thinking about anything at all"; he could influence them to do anything that he wanted and make them die or live, but "I like to keep them alive. If they do what they're told they keep alive." He would not expatiate upon how it was possible to achieve these things. With regard to number, I have mentioned the twenty hundred years that he is going to live. The number forty-two also had a special attraction for him. Thus he described a soldier injured in the First World War as having forty-two wounds between his legs; he could not describe how this number was counted. At a later point he stated that a milk separator had forty-two cups to it. He declared that he understood all about people's dreams, "just like a doctor", but he denied that he had any dreams himself.

His notions of birth and sex betrayed interesting features. Early in the testing he stated: "I understand a lot, cripples, ruptures and all that. If a baby is born crippled it came out of a crippled womb." Later he observed that he and the examiner were born different ways: he was born inside out but the examiner and all the other people in the world were born outside out; afterwards he modified this by saying that everybody was born inside out. These remarks were spontaneous. When questioned about conception, he denied that the male played any part in it. Women just became pregnant; he could not say why. He was asked to draw a figure of a man; then he was asked to draw the sex organs. He refused to do this, then and subsequently: "That would take too long to do. That takes a lot of time to do. I haven't time enough to think about that."

His concept of internal body-parts was investigated by getting him to draw a human figure and then insert the chief internal organs. No feature of special interest occurred in this performance. He was also asked a number of questions about inner organs. The curious answers here seemed to depend for the most part on ignorance rather than disturbance. He stated that the brain was in the back but not the front of the skull; under pressure as to what was behind the front of the skull he agreed that the brain must be there too. He declared that the lungs were concerned with chewing food, the kidneys with digestion, the liver with breathing. A matter of greater interest was his insistence that there were organs "in your posterior" other than the bowels or the sex organs; under pressure to explain what these were he withdrew the statement. Asked to say what there was behind the eyes he said, "There's danger behind them eyes more than what you understand. There's dark nights and other nights behind the eyes. Your head's not built the same as what mine is. There's a lot of difference. Your head's not been hurt at all. Mine's had more hurts than you'd ever understand. I've had the feeling of it and you've not." He stated that people were blue inside because their eyes were blue; people were not red inside like animals; if they were red inside there was something wrong with them and they would die.

With regard to external body-parts one or two points emerged in his sketches. The left ear was consistently drawn larger than the right; there was no such dyssymmetry in the other bilateral organs. In drawing a face he increased the size of the nostrils, with the observation, "must make the holes larger". He also spent some time elaborating the eyelashes, saying, "give him plenty of hair".

His Rorschach and Word-Association responses suggested an inquiry into his attitudes to colour. On the

Rorschach he exhibited the phenomenon of several pure colour responses, a characteristic behaviour of deteriorated schizophrenics. In the Word-Association there were some odd colour answers: thus to Blood he responded "Black", to Heart "Black" and to Death "Yellow". He was asked his preferences about the various colours; he stated that he liked blue and purple, greatly disliked yellow; about all other colours he merely said, "All right in its place". A number of colours were named to him and he was asked to exemplify each of them; his answers were: green for "beans", blue for "lilac", red for "paint", yellow for "a ruler", brown for "fruit", black for "a horse", grey for "wool", and white for "paper". A number of objects were named to him and he was asked to say what colour they were. Most of his answers were correct. One or two were remarkable: thus of blood he said, "it is all colours but generally it is black"; coal he said was blue: "if a coal marked your skin it would be a blue mark"; milk he also said was blue. His statement that people are blue inside has already been noted. These attitudes in relation to colour are of interest in connection with his refusal to do any painting. It may be added here that his colour-vision as tested by the Ishihara Test is completely normal.

Attempts to investigate his drawing under standard conditions were not successful, chiefly because he cannot sketch rapidly but elaborates his work slowly and with much effort. When he does a drawing he continues to fill in the whole sheet with matter irrelevant to the original subject but expressing his thought of the moment or the topic recently mentioned by the examiner. Mostly he talks as he works, less often he is silent. He finds it necessary to label with a written word many of the objects drawn. As I have said, three incidents were read to him which he was asked to illustrate. In two of these drawings he exhibited the phenomenon of spatial superposition of temporally successive events; in one of them he actually carried out the drawing, in the other a critical attitude emerged spontaneously and he stopped in the middle.

It will be evident that most of his behaviour when examined psychometrically can be described as demonstrating either inability to think conceptually or marked weakening in his capacity to do so. The purely perceptual continually invades the conceptual.

II

The psychiatric and psychometric study summarized above reveals a chronic schizophrenic, who exhibits some special features, which were discussed theoretically in the third chapter. To Freudian analysts the case seems to offer self-evident explanations. His meticulousness in drawing and his definite preoccupation with his posterior, his talk about it as soon as sex matters are mentioned, his constant worry about money, all invite the "anal erotic" commentary. His magic ceremonies carried out by producing the drawings fit in well with Freudian principles. On the other hand, the archaic appearance of his work would invite a Jungian analysis. Such interpretations, however, are lacking in sufficient proof, as I shall argue later.

One of the striking features of the patient's behaviour was the relation of everything to himself, and his constant comparison of himself to the examiner. This is a feature seen in some organic conditions as well as in children. It appears that the basic psychophysiological mechanism of it lies in the patient's attempt to experiment with his body-image, integrating it in comparison with the examiner. Such attempts are a normal phenomenon in children, because they are constantly shaping and re-building their body-image. Schizophrenics, however, are losing it, hence the patient's compensatory attempt to integrate his body-image through identification. His pre-occupation with his body-parts refers straightforwardly to body-image disturbances through which the outside world intrudes into the body. The disturbance is partly expressed in shift of the body-image in the anterior-posterior direction. Schilder found that in general the image of the brain is of something heavy in the region of the frontal bones. Mr. A.'s brain-image is at the occipital region, and so is his image of his testes. The disproportional representation of his left side appears to be dependent on the injury to his right arm and the fact that he has taught himself to make drawings with his left hand; because of this his left is over-emphasized and made dominant. Why this newly acquired leading hand shifted the body-image in a posterior direction could not be elucidated. His identifications with pictures in the test were similar to those of brain-injured cases; as Goldstein emphasized, such cases show a tendency to "physiognomic concreteness". One of Goldstein's patients described going through the door as "the door swallows me". Mr. A. shows similar tendencies as we saw in his responses to the picture-completion test and in the "keyhole" association response.

Such concreteness, which I shall treat more fully in Chapter 5, means that the function of abstract thinking is impaired. This is supported by further observations such as his association on "fur". As was said, it was not punning; it was due to the fact that at any moment words lose their conceptual value for such patients in a manner unsuspected by the hearer; they suddenly acquire a fundamentally purely perceptual value, or a mixture of perceptual and conceptual qualities. It might well be that his perseveration is another expression of a merely perceptual value of words, which are just meaninglessly repeated.

Animism as an expression of disturbed body-imagery and impaired conceptual thinking is well instanced by Mr. A.'s remarks on movement, when he indicated that all movements, human or mechanical, have the same motivation behind them.

All those evaluations, however, become more evident when studied in connection with his drawings, of which only three will be reproduced here. The first one is "The Derby", the second "The Old River" and the third "The Horses and Flooding" (Figs. 11, 12 and 13). In general they show the typical schizophrenic features;

meticulous over-elaboration of details, playful irre-
levancies such as the butterfly in "The Horses and
Flooding", "writing in", etc., with mannerisms in the
lettering. "The Derby" is interesting because its content
demands a spatial representation of a temporal event.
His technique in solving this is twofold. The horses, when
lined up, are superimposed on one another as if each
were transparent, so that the whole line can be seen.
After the start he represents them twice again, when
running and at the finish. These three representations of
the runners are deliberate, because at the start there is no
hot air steaming from the horses' nostrils, but later this is
carefully represented to indicate that the course is coming
to a finish. Thus, it appears, spatial representation of
duration presented little that is problematic to Mr. A.;
this might point to the fact that his time-space system has
lost its proper interrelation. In the "Old River" all
figures are himself; when it was pointed out to him that
he could not be eight times in the same landscape at a
given moment, he argued that he could. He also argued
that the rider on horseback was himself too, but "that
happened at another time". He was asked why then it
should be put into the same picture; he stated that "all
things happen all the time". It appeared that in discussing his pictures his idea of time somewhat contra-
dicted the psychometric findings; it was a time relation
of spatial character. The difference here probably depends on the fact that the psychometric examination
pinned Mr. A. down to precise statements and induced
critical realistic attitudes, whereas in discussing the drawings he was free to follow his preferred phantastic modes
of thought. The disturbed spatial experience is also expressed in faulty configuration (Gestaltung); these pictures have no delineation in relation to the surrounding
space—they are completely lacking in spatial unity. Even
in "The Derby", where the oval shape of the race-course
would have automatically given a closed shape, it remained open; questions about this only led to long,
irrelevant discussions with Mr. A.

As it was emphasized, disturbed time-space relations are interconnected with disturbances of conceptual thinking. These disturbances are well exemplified in the pictures. The mixture of conceptual elements, the "writing in", is one of them. More striking are these mixtures of conceptual and concretistic representation in the figures themselves. For instance, "The Horses" is primarily representation; two horses actually were in a field. The River Medway had flooded the field and the horses had nothing to eat. Hence Mr. A. (in the top corner of the picture) brought them hay to feed them. But to give more food to them he drew a milk bottle between the heads of the two horses, so that for certain they should not starve. The horses, however, are not produced only as he saw them existing; though they are standing on all four limbs, the horse-shoes are drawn in on each hoof with nails and all, because he knows they had shoes—horses in general are shod. Similarly in the case of the trees, though their appearance is only trunk and crown, he always draws the roots as well, because root, trunk and crown are essential parts of a tree. Aestheticians have drawn attention to the fact that oriental artists do not paint the actual appearance only but the essence of the thing as well; consequently in most of their pictures it is not *a* tree depicted but *the* tree. Similarly Mr. A.'s pictures show a mixture of reproduction of the existent and the essential, the reproduction of perceptual reality and also of its abstracted concept. These types of symbol are the ones which have induced Jung's adherents to assume a universality of symbols. In some primitive cultures the "skeleton drawing", or "X-ray drawing", is a frequent way of pictorial representation. In fact, Mr. A.'s fish, as in "The Old River", is almost identical with drawings of the Kakadu tribe as reproduced in B. Spencer's book. As I have said, primitives are in process of conceptualizing, whereas schizophrenics are deteriorating from abstract thinking to a level which is similar to some pre-literate thinking, since it is a mixture of concepts and concretistic elements. Hence the similarity between the pictorial expressions.

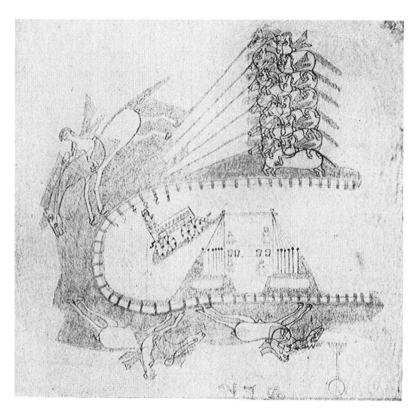

Fig. 11. 'Derby'

face p. 86

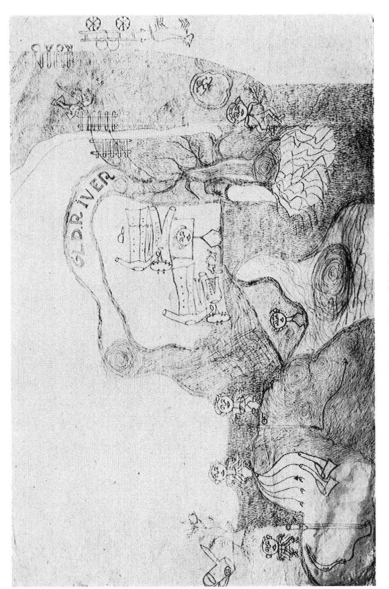

Fig. 12. 'The Old River'

The body-image disturbances are well appreciated when one compares "The Old River" with "The Derby". In the latter all figures, including the barmaids in the beer-tent, fill their clothes well; they all have substantial bodies. Mr. A. himself, however, in "The Old River" is merely a faint skeleton held together only by clothing. When, after fishing, he undresses, the clothing, like a live thing, lies on the ground leaving him a pathetic lemur, shivering; and in the water his arms become dissolved. When discussing this picture, as I have indicated, he admitted that all the figures were himself, and he stated that he *was* thin, adding that the little figure in the circle "is me outside the world". After much discussion he spontaneously returned to this picture and said that he could be himself and everything else as well, and that the picture started by himself being outside the world. This seems to be an attempt to demarcate himself somehow, as otherwise he would be one with the whole world, thus developing an animistic belief. He not only stated that he was every figure in the picture, but that he was the whole world and the tree in the picture as well. He commented on this, saying: "I am the tree as well; you can be all these things. You eat yeast, which comes from the tree, so you become a tree. I am a tree and I am all the people in the world." He re-emphasized that he was a tree and a person and all the world. This short quotation might have come from a pre-literate native, the animism is so marked. It strikingly expressed the loss of body demarcations and dissolution of the body in the temporal and spatial surroundings. One should regard this as chiefly a cognitive phenomenon. The outlook of the schizophrenic patient approximates in this respect to what has often been observed in very young children. The spatial boundaries between the body and the outside world are extremely tenuous; there is deficiency in the conceptual ordering of space. The conceptual ordering of time is also deficient; there is no schema of past events; the distinction between what is past and what is present loses its sharpness.

It seems that when he was confronted with his pictures

7

relevant material was easily obtained. This brings me to the final question, what function these pictures had for him, whether they had magic value? When asked why he did them, he gave on various occasions identical answers. He said that those pictures "prove that I am here", i.e. that he exists at present. All the things in the pictures *did* happen, and by depicting his past life he feels assured of his existence in the present—and as it was made certain, present was literally meant and not future or eternity. Thus those pictures fulfilled for him an absolutely vital function; they kept him, so to say, alive. I have remarked schizophrenics often pinch themselves or inflict other injuries to themselves, such as pulling out their hair, actions which make them experience the reality of their body. Schizophrenic paintings are similar actions in a creative sense; Mr. A. confirmed that through drawing he could experience and maintain his existence.

To sum it up, the motivating factors in his drawings were: weakening of his conceptual thinking, which was also ascertained psychometrically; disturbance of his body-image, which was also evident clinically; and disturbance of time-space relations, evidenced in the pictures and supported clinically. His "animism" was interconnected with those factors; the interpretative concept of "magic" was not necessary for elucidation of his actions. It should be re-emphasized that the evaluation outlined is descriptive and not speculative. One is aware, however, that these biological factors are not the total motivation of schizophrenic art; neither do they answer the problem of why Mr. A. is creative and other schizophrenic patients are not.

V

THE NATURE OF PSYCHOTIC ART

The cognitive aspect—Spearman's theory and criticism of it— Goldstein's approach—Similarities between psychotic and non-psychotic art products.

THE PRECEDING CHAPTERS have argued that the peculiarities and special features of schizophrenic painting depend primarily on cognitive abnormalities in the patient. One basic motivation leading to the spontaneous and abundant production of pictures by schizophrenics is, according to the evidence I have adduced, their attempt to adjust themselves to an altered apprehension of reality. The disturbances of thinking in schizophrenia have been viewed from a psycho-physiological standpoint with particular attention to the phenomenon of the body-image, an approach which I believe to be well founded in biology. In analysing the body-image as a conceptual schema we have seen how closely it is linked with the concepts of space and time; and we have seen that disturbances in the concepts of space and time can be induced experimentally by the administration of mescalin and that the disturbances so occasioned are accompanied by visual hallucinations. I also pointed out that disordering in the conceptual systems of space and time leads inevitably to a general disorganization of conceptual thinking.

My previous discussion has touched on the number of apparent resemblances between schizophrenic painting and modern pictorial art. This apparent similarity has been seized on by many commentators on modern art who do not sympathize with its development. It is frequently mentioned by visitors to art exhibitions, who have not trained themselves to appreciate the work of modern painters or who are deficient in the capacity for aesthetic enjoyment. But sometimes the similarity is also accepted by present-day artists and those who are in sympathy with modern painting. Schizophrenic art products are then regarded as having aesthetic status equivalent to that of paintings by normal artists; the fact of mental illness is considered either to be irrelevant or else as a stimulus to satisfactory work. Those who take the latter view have usually had little opportunity of examining much psychotic painting; moreover, they have probably not formulated at all clearly for themselves the characteristics which distinguish pictorial production as an aesthetic activity. It must be emphasized very strongly that when large numbers of art products by normal modern artists and by schizophrenic patients are carefully scrutinized and compared, the resemblances are found to be apparent and superficial, the differences fundamental and profound. The work of normal artists reveals a deliberate re-structuring of presented reality into complex patterns or relations of form and colour. The work of schizophrenics reveals no such deliberate and complex restructuring but on the contrary a general lack of structure, a disintegration of perceptual relations and a dissolution of concepts. The apparent similarity is due to the fact that both in modern and in schizophrenic pictorial activity the relations of presented reality are radically altered; in normal painting before the modern epoch the alterations were usually less radical. In the painting of modern artists—this is the basic, all-important difference—the radical alteration is one of re-organization, in the work of schizophrenics it is one of disorganization. The patterning of normal artists is complex, many-sided and systematic; the patterning of schizophrenics is chiefly disorganized and unsystematic.

I have purposely set out the difference once more, in sharply opposed terms, whereas in fact there exist intermediate cases in which schizophrenic illness interacts with artistic ability and training. Such cases as these have reinforced the supposition that trends in modern art are related to the phenomena of mental illness. A few normal artists develop an overt schizophrenic disorder and under its influence their work steadily disintegrates; I have discussed one such instance in Chapter 2. No doubt, too, a certain number of apparently normal artists, like some apparently normal individuals in other professions, have latent schizophrenic tendencies and exhibit underlying schizophrenic modes of thought; such tendencies can be detected in their work by the observer skilled enough in discrimination. This is true only of a small minority of artists. It also happens that some schizophrenic patients have high innate artistic abilities and sufficient training to give their work a genuine artistic character, though not sufficient to constitute them artists. The work of such patients has, besides its psychotic features, real aesthetic value of greater or less degree and can be appreciated in the same manner as normal art. Despite all intermediate possibilities, however, the general distinction between normal modern art and the pictorial activity of the mentally diseased is clear and outstanding.

This stress on the relational character of normal art and on thinking disorders as the primary determinant of schizophrenic pictorial production demands a more extended discussion of art as a cognitive phenomenon. My view implies a close interconnection between art and conceptional thinking. Both may be described as human peculiarities. Man's capacity for conceptual thinking must be regarded as the capacity which most distinguishes him from the lower animals and the one on which his mastery of his environment essentially depends. The barest rudiments of conceptual thinking can be detected below the human level in the recognition of similarities, in the isolation of aspects and in other behaviours shown in problem-solving situations by animals which possess a well-defined cortex, but it does not require demonstration that man possesses these capacities in a measure far transcending that of any other animal and that he alone is capable of dealing with the possible as well as the actual. Artistic production in any degree of development is likewise an exclusively human characteristic. Nothing parallel to it is evident in the infra-human mammalian series. Certain activities in birds, it is true, such as the displays associated with mating and the rituals which go with a change of duties in the care of the young, may be a parallel specialized development of the same basic tendency in animal nature which is latent in the infra-human mammals; artistic development then, like colour-discrimination, paternal care and quasi-permanent mating, might be considered as a concealed possibility in the animal organism which evolutionary processes bring to the surface in widely separated zoological classes. The complex, relational character of artistic production in man, however, makes it quite distinctive of the human species and at the same time indicates how closely it is involved with conceptional thinking.

Consideration of art as a cognitive phenomenon at once raises the problem of why certain individuals are able to produce pictorial art while others are not. In dealing with psychotic art it raises the problem of why only some schizophrenics paint or draw. These matters are not, of course, purely cognitive; orectic questions of drive and motivations are likewise concerned. But here, I believe, the cognitive aspect is the more important. One is led to inquire what cognitive difference can be found between the artistic and the non-artistic in pictorial art. First it is necessary to make a general analysis of the cognitive activities and capacities involved in aesthetic drawing or painting. Four independent aspects can be distinguished: unlearned motor and perceptual aptitudes, learned skills of craftsmanship and technique, relational thinking and aesthetic creativity. As a basis for this discussion, especially

of the motor and perceptual skills, it will be desirable to
outline the ontogenetic development of drawing in the
child. This has been investigated chiefly in America, but Sir
Cyril Burt, who has ably summarized the American conclusions, has verified that in general they can be applied
also to children in Great Britain. Essentially similar
accounts have been given by Lowenfeld and many others.

Burt notes that the development of drawing in children
is a matter of spasmodic growth with unexpected meta-
morphoses. The progression shows changes in kind as
well as in degree; there is a movement from one unique
phase to another through a series of transformations. He
distinguishes seven main stages, each of which glides im-
perceptibly into the next; within several of these stages he
distinguishes sub-stages. In the early stages up to the age
of 5 the interest is motor rather than visual; there is
little control by sight. To begin with, movements of the
arm are dominant; gradually movements of the wrist
come to dominate movements of the arm and in turn are
dominated by finger-movements. The earliest stage is that
of scribble; the child begins with purposeless pencillings
enjoyed for the sake of movement and passes through
phases of purposive pencilling, imitative pencilling and
localized pencilling to a point where activity is limited to
a single movement instead of rhythmic oscillations. The
rate and succession of development is modified by instruction at home or at school. The child names his products
in various ways, but his interest tends to focus more and
more exclusively on representing the human form. This
fact is clearly correlated with that building up of the body-
schema to which I have referred in Chapter 4. The human
form is first represented with juxtaposition rather than
synthesis of parts and then at the stage of descriptive
symbolism develops into a crude symbolic schema. The
schema varies from child to child but each child sticks to
the same schema for man and woman and for animals,
if he represents them. Both at this stage and at the subsequent one, which Burt calls descriptive realism, the child
is thinking of the generic type, not the model. Perceptual

interest is in the background; most children do not look at the model they are drawing, a few look at it once only. At this stage, of course, the process of concept formation is still in full swing. During this period, about the age of seven, the important change from full-face to profile representation occurs; some children go through a phase in which they produce hybrids between the two incompatible aspects. Round about the ages of 9 to 10 there occurs a sharp metamorphosis. Motor skill and representative technique improve immensely and interest shifts to detailed perceptual observation. The child traces the drawings of others and draws spontaneously from nature. He begins to represent landscapes and particular individuals. Representation moves from a two-dimensional to a three-dimensional sub-phase. In the pre-pubertal period, usually about the age of 13, there ensues a stage of repression, in which drawings often show an apparent deterioration or regression. Conventional designs are produced but the human figure is avoided. Burt remarks that obscure intellectual and emotional factors underlie this repression but suggests that increased self-criticism, more careful perceptual observation, and a transference of interest to expression through language may be the chief determinants. After this phase of repression the majority of children never draw again. In a few, however, there is an artistic revival in early adolescence when for the first time genuine aesthetic activity appears. Drawings tell a story, or, if instruction has favoured it, demonstrate principles of formal design; when human figures are represented they approximate to the portraits of the professional artist.

As already noted, teaching considerably modifies the progression of stages I have just described. It has traditionally been the endeavour of teachers to develop the child's perceptual observations as early and fully as possible and to encourage the drawings of various objects in addition to the human figure. Modern teachers of art have emphasized and encouraged creative ability rather than motor and perceptual skills. They believe that the phase of pre-pubertal repression need not inevitably ensue and have done everything to tide it over or eliminate it. It is their contention that the motor and perceptual capacities and the creative ability on which the production of aesthetically satisfying art depends are latent in every human being and can be made manifest by skilful instruction and encouragement. There is no doubt that this is true. But it is also true that great individual differences exist and that some persons have potentialities much in excess of the majority.

So far as motor capacities are concerned the existence of marked individual differences among children in the efficiency of their performance is implied at a number of points in Burt's account. He does not, however, discuss them very explicitly except in connection with mental deficiency. The fact of considerable individual differences in sheer motor capacity to draw can easily be verified by asking a number of adults who have had no training to sketch a man or a cat or to copy some form or figure. Quite independently of perceptual and conceptual aspects the results vary from the highly effective to the grossly inadequate. In fact, one can say that a fair number of individuals have a distinct disability in this direction. Teachers of drawing likewise agree that both children and adults vary markedly in the speed with which they acquire the necessary motor skills and in the level they finally reach. The variation almost certainly depends on innate differences in motor aptitude. It shows some relationship to general intelligence, but as Burt indicates not a single or linear one. That the relationship is not very close is suggested by fairly numerous cases in which motor disability in drawing co-exists with high efficiency in dealing with abstract verbal or numerical material. Possession of this innate motor aptitude in a considerable degree is without doubt an essential component in pictorial production, aesthetic and non-aesthetic. It is a necessary condition of the fact that some people become pictorial artists while others do not. Its occurrence in low or high degree would also appear to be a determinant of the fact that only some schizophrenics draw or paint. While, however, it is a necessary condition of pictorial production it is very far from being a sufficient one, as I shall shortly argue.

Most artists and persons who display artistic talents are found to have drawn well in childhood, that is to say, they possessed in high measure the motor aptitude necessary for effective representation on paper. There appear to be some exceptions, however, and the converse is not true; many people who draw well in childhood show no artistic abilities in later life and in certain cases are even not very effective in the motor skills of drawing. These circumstances, as Burt indicates, make it extremely difficult to diagnose special artistic powers before puberty; the fact that motor skill is only one component of artistic ability complicates the situation still more. Even in the most precocious, Burt states it is not possible to predict artistic talent before the calendar age of eleven. Nevertheless, examination of the life-history of professional artists indicates that their steps were first set in this direction by the realization that they possessed in an unusual degree the motor skill for pictorial representation, the satisfaction this gave them and the approbation it won from others. That some possessing this skill never become artists depends partly on environmental factors, lack of opportunity and encouragement or the like, but mainly on deficiency in other components of artistic ability, relational thinking and creativity.

The conditions underlying differences in the motor aptitude for drawing have not been very satisfactorily analysed or investigated. Educational psychologists have inquired into the cognate problem of the movements employed in handwriting, but so far as drawing is concerned their interest has lain principally in the training of perceptual observation and in the encouragement of creative activity. In the vocational guidance of adolescents no elaborate analysis of what is involved by the ability to draw has been required, since an individual's success in an artistic career can be most easily and reliably predicted by examining his actual products.

It is evident that the motor aptitude for drawing belongs to the class of manual dexterities. The general characteristics of these have been investigated by a number of workers, especially in this country, by F. M. Earle, F. Gaw and J. Cox; their results agree more or less completely. All investigators concur that manual dexterity is quite distinct from mechanical aptitude and nearly all that manual dexterity is specific to a particular task, that is, that there are manual dexterities and not a general capacity of manual dexterity. Earle and Gaw analyse any given manual dexterity into two components—first, a co-ordination of the separate activities of different muscle systems, brought about by the subordination of these separate movements to the purpose of the activity as a whole, and secondly, a general bodily "set", peculiar to the person carrying out the movement. The first component they regard as having its physical basis in the connections of the nervous system; it is influenced by practice, fatigue, drugs, emotional excitement and the like. The second component depends on structure, length of limbs, muscular development and so on; this factor of " set " varies from one process to the other and is probably responsible for the high independence of the abilities involved in manual dexterities. Earle and Gaw discuss classes of purposive manual movements; drawing is nearest to their third class, those movements in which accuracy is the chief factor and rate of movement is comparatively unimportant.

The studies of F. N. Freeman on the manual dexterities in handwriting help to explain those involved in drawing. The writing and drawing dexterities both centre on directing with the hand the movements of an implement such as a pencil or pen. Both are complex organizations of many elementary or simple movements. The most basic dexterity of all is that of separating the first and second fingers in their action from the third and fourth so that the implement is grasped between the thumb and first two fingers while the third and fourth support the weight of the hand. It is a familiar fact that the capacity to place the thumb against the tip of the fingers in grasping an object is one of those distinctive of man. The more primitive form of grasping, which appears first in the child and is the only form seen in the other primates, is that of folding the four fingers about the object without using the thumb. Besides the dexterity of grasping, other important dexterities involved in the process of writing and drawing are various movements of the arm joints, especially shoulder, fore-arm and wrist movements. As already noted, the progression is from emphasis on arm-movements to emphasis on wrist-movements and from the latter to emphasis on finger-movements. Sometimes it is stated that the progression is from fundamental or phylogenetically old movements to accessory or phylogenetically recent movements; the fundamental movements are sometimes identified with movements of the large muscles and sometimes with movements concerned with the trunk or parts of limbs next to the trunk. The empirical investigations, however, indicate that the progression cannot be satisfactorily described in these terms. As the child advances in its capacity to write or draw, the basic component dexterities are built up into a total large movement which is rhythmical and regular. Besides the manual dexterities, adjustments of the eye and of the body posture are integrated into the total movement. The process of learning to write or draw in its motor aspect is one of selecting appropriate movements, inhibiting contrary movements, and co-ordinating those selected into a rhythmical chronological system. Both in writing and drawing the movements improve markedly from the age of six to that of sixteen in rapidity, steadiness and precision; the improvement takes place in irregular phases. At all ages of childhood there are striking individual differences in the capacity to execute the movements dexterously, and these differences are also strikingly evident in adults.

Although in the first stage of learning to draw the emphasis is chiefly motor, this shifts at a fairly early point to emphasis on the perceptual and conceptual aspects of

what is represented. All three aspects are, of course, interwoven in the mature performance; their separation is
artificial and usually only of theoretical interest. Nevertheless cases of discrepancy where motor skills are of high
degree but accompanied by no aesthetic creativity and
vice versa indicate that the aspects are separable at times.

The perceptual aspects of drawing do not require an
extended discussion. Innate differences in this regard are
overlaid by the effects of training at various levels. The
essential perceptual element in drawing is the recognition
of form, gained through active exploration, and inter-
acting at all times with the motor representation of form.
This recognition is closely linked with symbolic and
generalizing behaviour. Perception develops as an organization of impression and includes processes of analysis
and synthesis. For the most part accurate and detailed
observation of perceptual relationships is a function of
intellectual capacity in conjunction with training, but
there are individual differences of general intelligence.
Besides specific differences in sensory acuity some persons
observe concrete details better than they observe emotional
states and reactions, some the reverse. Some individuals
introduce interpretation into their perceptual observations much more than others. A few people of very high
ability are astonishingly weak in their observation of
concrete spatial relationships.

The teaching of craftsmanship in drawing is essentially
the same process at all levels. It differs chiefly in complexity from the early efforts with young children to the
advanced instruction at the school of art. The emphasis,
of course, may vary between accuracy of representation
and the production of satisfying formal relations; as I
have already argued, the latter is the necessary condition
of art and in recent decades has mainly been stressed.
The acquisition of craftsmanship is principally a question
of mastering effective representative and suggestive techniques—perspective, black and white shading, use of
shadows, recession of masses, employment of colour in
terms of light, and so on—and of learning the processes

of formal design—composition, selection, elimination, modification. The representative and suggestive techniques can probably be taught to anyone, though persons with a high motor aptitude for drawing and with a good capacity for accurate perceptual observation are likely to master them more quickly and effectively than those who are deficient in these respects. The processes of formal design can be taught only in part; they are too much involved with relational thinking and aesthetic creativity to be mastered in any effective degree except by a gifted minority. It is not difficult to find individuals who have marked skill so far as the representative and suggestive techniques are concerned and even in the principles of formal design, inasmuch as these can be reduced to rule of thumb, but who are exceedingly deficient in aesthetic creativity. Such people may be called craftsmen as opposed to creative artists.

At this point it will be useful to interpolate a neurological discussion of the bases of motor aptitude in drawing and the higher capacities which are necessary in the constitution of an artist. It has been found that slight damage to the motor cortical area is followed on the opposite side of the body by clumsiness of finger-movements, leading to a disturbed performance. Such a disturbance is essentially a motor phenomenon with little relevance to higher performances. Differences in motor aptitude for drawing can plausibly be related to structure or functional difference in this cortical area. They may also be related to another phenomenon which seems especially applicable to instances of people possessing high capacity for perceptual observation, relational thinking, and aesthetic creativity but grossly deficient in the capacity to express pictorially their creative schemata. This condition is that of ideomotor apraxia, which appears without involvement of the motor system proper. The patient loses his ability to perform intended movements but spontaneously or by reflexes can carry out old habitual motor patterns, often with perseveration. Ideomotor apraxia depends on a lesion in the region of the brain where the temporal, parietal and occipital lobes meet. In this region of the leading hemisphere, especially in the supramarginal and angular gyrus, the most refined functions appear to be located. Visual agnosia, body-image disturbances, aphasia, loss of orientation in space, and ideomotor apraxia result from lesions of these centres. Furthermore, Schilder has reported that lesions of the dominant supramarginal gyrus result in an asymbolia for pain; the patients feel pain but are unable to symbolize their experience of it. Another neurological observation is that lesions of the angular gyrus not only result in aphasia but produce a situation in which the patient can draw from memory but cannot draw present complex objects. I do not propose to enumerate more fully the symptomatology of this region of the brain which in phylogenetic perspective is more unique than the so-called frontal lobes, but the few examples that I have quoted demonstrate convincingly that symbolic formation should be correlated with this area.

From the physiological viewpoint, as expected, these observations contradict a dichotomy of reception and expression. One cannot state when symbolic formation ends and symbolic expression begins. The idea of performance can only be divorced theoretically from the performance itself. In other words, the artist's ability to re-structure reality cannot be analysed into two distinct processes of symbolic formulation and expression, since both are highly interwoven. Artistic creation is more than motor and perceptual skills; it has always an ideational component as well. If such a comparison might be permissible, the difference between the artist and the non-artist who is appreciative of art lies in an ideational apraxia of the non-artist. Another interesting reflection on the structural and functional link just mentioned is that the body-image, spatial orientation, symbolic formulation, plans of skilled movements, etc., are all condensed in this area. At this point, it will be convenient to discuss more fully the relation between artistic production on the one hand and cerebral structure and functioning on the other.

Interest in the problems of brain injury has been renewed since the operation of leucotomy has been used in the treatment of mental disorders. This operation aims at inflicting bilateral symmetrical injury to the prefrontal lobes, by undercutting fibres which constitute the white matter of the prefrontal part of the brain. Opinions on the advisability, technique, indications and evaluations of this treatment vary, but there seems to be a fair agreement on its action in a broad sense. By this induced injury a new symptomatology is produced, which balances with the pre-existing mental symptoms, and brings about a social adjustment in the patient. We need not discuss in detail all the problems of this empirical treatment, which probably induces cognitive, conative and affective changes in the patient's personality, but a few points are of interest because they are relevant to artistic creativity.

Previously I have quoted Schilder's work, pointing out that the posterior part of the brain might be responsible for the symbolic formulation of pain; it has been found, however, that a similar event takes place after leucotomy. I have also pointed to the fact that the idea of an action corresponds to the functions of the posterior part of the brain; on the other hand, the symptoms arising from prefrontal leucotomy have been evaluated as a loss of foresight, a loss of the ultimate weighing of actions. Apathy has been looked upon as a symptom of various diseased brain centres, yet diminished conation and emotional blunting have been described as typical sequels of bilateral prefrontal leucotomy. These and several other symptoms might support the hypothesis, suggested on other grounds as well, that the localization of function to a certain part of the brain is only *more or less* correct, and that a function is always a result of the inter-action of several "centres". Nevertheless, a fairly well controlled interference with a certain part of the brain allows observation of the induced symptoms, even if the explanations may differ. It also gives an opportunity of correlating structural alterations to psychophysiological events and so ultimately of studying injury to the brain in relation to artistic activity.

Of the large number of studies of leucotomy, only a few deal with leucotomy and artistic activity. Professor Freeman had a patient who painted pictures of real merit, yet after leucotomy he "came down to earth and his creative urge was soon extinguished".* Later, in a paper given together with Watts, Freeman speculated on the factors which might affect creativity. Creative work, he concluded, is based on phantasy, which demands foresight: "no work of art can be created without visualizing the effect before it is undertaken". In leucotomized patients the structure mediating phantasy is destroyed; hence creativity proper is lost for them. Apart from the attempt to localize phantasy in the prefrontal lobe, the shortcoming of this speculation lies in the fact that creativity involves very many more factors than those singled out by Freeman. E. Hutton and M. Bassett corrected this shortcoming; they recognized four factors in creative activity: (1) imagination; (2) emotional motives and associated judgements of value; (3) technical knowledge and practical activity; (4) sustained effort and persistent application. They found that leucotomy in the first six weeks after the operation alters these factors: creative imagination is much reduced and made almost non-existent; emotional motives and associated judgements of value are weakened and there is a decrease in effort and application. Thus they concluded, like Freeman, that there is a decrease in creativity following bilateral prefrontal leucotomy. Although these authors themselves criticized the psychometric methods which they employed to verify their statements, their argument was to a certain degree based on a case that exhibited creativity prior to operation. Alas! the patient was a Hungarian poet and this makes their conclusion the less applicable when discussing pictorial art.

My own investigations, before those of the authors I have quoted, posed the problems differently. In the first place, 8 per cent. of my operated case material took to drawing shortly after the operation, but the urge to

* Personally communicated.

8

continue disappeared at the time when definite improvement became manifest. Previous investigators found, however, that only 2 per cent. of schizophrenics produce spontaneous drawings; thus I am inclined to think that there *is* a creative spell following the operation, though my speculations on the psycho-pathological nature of this induced creativity may be controversial. Secondly, my observations were related to schizophrenics who showed peculiarities in their mental life and in their pictorial activities, as described in previous chapters. Now it has been observed that the artistic products of patients with brain injury of various localizations exhibit a certain orderliness, a tendency to avoid empty spaces, and a perseverative trend, together with a disordered choice of colour. There are changes of configuration: there is a tendency to curves instead of angles, figures may be contracted or expanded and elongated. Thus the pictorial activity of patients with brain injury resembles in some respects schizophrenic pictorial activity. The differences, however, I found in a more marked disturbance of the figure-background relation, in more pronounced disintegration in the system of relations and in a very apparent *horror vacui*. On the other hand, the postoperative appearances were more often as follows: the patient painted in one corner of the sheet of paper objects without any relation to one another: a dress, birds flying, a bell, four dots. As the post-operative period progressed, the paintings moved more into the centre of the paper. Two weeks after operation the same patient made a drawing of a woman jumping from a jumping board; in the sky were some birds and beneath some blue dots; thus the discrete parts became interrelated one with another; the picture became an organized whole. This is a more striking example, since at other times the picture appeared as chaotic conglomerates of schizophrenic and brain-injured expressions.

The importance of these observations in relation to formal appearances is that fundamentally they are similar to the results of less specified brain injuries. They indicate that any cerebral catastrophe results in a universal reaction, as seen in pictorial expression; thus they give yet another indication of the importance of the structural relations of functional integrity. They also indicate that to search for a cerebral centre of artistic talent is useless and that it is the total brain, in particular its function, which has to be studied in this connection.

To return to the psychological problems, the whole burden of my discussion so far has been to emphasize the components of relational and conceptual thinking involved in aesthetic pictorial activity. The classic analysis of the cognitive processes concerned in the production and enjoyment of pictorial art is that of C. Spearman. He distinguishes five aspects in pictorial art—truth, beauty, emotionality, exaggeration and self-expression—and relates all these primarily to his third neogenetic principle, the creation of correlative fundaments. More remotely they depend on his other principles of experience and relations, and most basically of all, he states, probably on emotion and sub-conscious activity. He decisively rejects the view that to explain aesthetic creativity one must assume the existence of supernatural powers in the artist. Besides relating the five aspects of art to his qualitative principles of neogenesis, Spearman also relates them to his quantitative principles—constancy of output, retentivity, fatigue, conative control and primordial potencies. The aspect of truth he views as a relation of likeness between the painting and what is represented. So far as the aspect of beauty is concerned Spearman notes that marked divergences of view exist on what is meant by beauty, and he then analyses the variable carefully in terms of energy and his five quantitative principles. Constancy of output implies that everything irrelevant to the aim must be abandoned; energy tends to adopt a unified mode of distribution and the aesthetic interest of the picture must be adopted to such a unifocal distribution of energy. Retentivity demands that there should be repetition in the painting, patterns and relational systems of varying complexity, built up into general structures whose form may be that of the circle, the ellipse, the pyramid, parallel lines and so on. Fatigue on the contrary demands that there should be variety besides repetition, difference as well as likeness, multiplicity in unity, leading to harmony, rhythm and balance. Conative control functions in art by indicating how far the flow of energy is perfect; the individual enjoying art bases his evaluation not on the absolute amount of the stream of energy but on the ratio of this to the effort he makes. By primordial potencies Spearman denotes irregularities between the mental powers of different individuals; in pictorial art these are displayed in the fact that a product which leads to perfect energizing in the sophisticated expert may occasion only confusion and pain in others. Spearman touches on the cultural, historical and geographical differences in the production and appreciation of pictorial art by noting that if a person has adopted a particular view and finds paintings done otherwise he will be thwarted in his conation and his energizing will be vitiated because the system of relations does not accord with expectation. He also follows Sir Charles Myers in distinguishing different attitudes in the appreciation of art, a passive attitude of contemplation and an active pursuit of similarities and other relations. Spearman believes that pleasure is obtained chiefly by the active perception of relations, but Myers holds the view that both the active and passive attitudes have their rewards.

The aspect of emotionality Spearman relates to his principle of retentivity; the principle of fatigue is involved only to a slight extent. The emotions evoked are make-believe ones which come by association. The other aspects of exaggeration and self-expression he does not so closely link to the distribution of energy. He notes that when the natural appearance is transcended it is usually a process of exaggeration; this process has limits and if carried far becomes caricature. Self-expression is largely a question of individual differences and personal style. Spearman distinguishes four sub-aspects here; technical differences in the use and application of implements and materials; differences in breadth—a tendency to multiplication of details is characteristic of some artists, a general simplifying tendency is characteristic of others; individual stylization; and personal phantasies which in an extreme form find their match in those of the schizophrenic.

There can be no doubt that Spearman's analysis is searching and illuminating. I am in thorough agreement with his treatment of artistic production and appreciation as being chiefly cognitive, relational activities. I would incline to attach less importance than he does to the aspects of truth and emotionality and much more to the aspects of exaggeration, regarded rather as re-structuring, and beauty, regarded as a patterning of relations. The latter two aspects seem to me the necessary constituents of aesthetic activity; the others are merely possible concomitants. While Spearman's account is so fundamental, it still needs to be amplified and verified by empirical inquiries, particularly in regard to its biological foundations and the impact upon it of cultural factors. Spearman seems to have relied almost exclusively on introspective analysis in this matter without experimental checks. His explanation in terms of the distribution of energy is entirely speculative. By energy, of course, he denotes his concept of "mental energy"; it has been abundantly demonstrated by a number of writers, notably Burt and Godfrey Thomson, that the concept of mental energy is either meaningless or a deceptive metaphor. His principle of fatigue is contrary to several findings in experimental psychology. While Spearman touches on cultural factors in relation to art he gives them inadequate weight; and one may note that few individuals trained in the appreciation of pictorial art during the past half century or more would agree that many of the examples chosen by Spearman are aesthetically satisfying; his standards seem to be those of a period rather distant in the nineteenth century. The most important deficiency in Spearman's account, however, is that it does not adequately explain why some individuals are aesthetically creative and others are not. Besides the instances of people intellectually able to re-structure presented reality into a pattern and disposed to do so but unable to express their re-structuring effectively owing to weakness in motor aptitude, there are also individuals with high ability in relational thinking and a high degree of motor aptitude for drawing who despite this cannot produce aesthetically creative work. Such persons are usually excellent photographic copyists and can produce highly effective anatomical and botanical drawings and so on. Spearman would seem to imply that aesthetic creativity depends solely on high ability in relational thinking and that difference in this regard between individuals of apparently equivalent intellectual capacity springs entirely from environmental conditioning or temperamental tendencies. Undoubtedly the chances of environmental stimulation and such orectic factors as emotional responsiveness and expressivity are important determinants here. I am strongly of the opinion, however, that a part equally important is played by basic, innate differences in cognitive attitude and approach which bring it about that people deal with relations in different ways and vary considerably in their capacity to deal with different kinds of relations. Spearman suggests differences in conative attitudes so far as appreciation is concerned and differences in breadth of approach so far as execution is concerned. These attitudinal differences, especially the cognitive ones, seem to me to require much more extended investigation and analysis.

A noteworthy extension of Spearman's aesthetic theory has been made by H. J. Eysenck, who has endeavoured to remove some of its weaknesses and to relate it to the concept of Good Gestalt. He emphasizes that the problems of aesthetics are essentially problems of perceptual processes and that the laws of beauty can be reduced to problems of perception. So he defines the beautiful in its formal aspect in terms of "order multiplied by complexity", where order is a simplifying and complexity a

differentiating principle. Dealing with aesthetic appreciation he states that intercorrelational analysis has demonstrated the existence of a general component so that
persons aesthetically appreciative of visual stimuli are
also aesthetically appreciative of auditory stimuli, performance and so on. This general component, named the
T-factor, is correlated with intelligence to a small but
statistically significant extent. Analysis of correlations also
shows the existence of a bipolar group factor in aesthetic
appreciation related to introversion and extraversion, and
of specific factors related to individual peculiarities.
Eysenck formulates a general law of aesthetic appreciation, with three corollaries, in terms of the distribution
of energy in the nervous system. He abandons Spearman's principle of fatigue and attempts to avoid the
difficulties occasioned by the concept "mental energy"
by equating it with neural energy. There can be no
doubt that Eysenck is right in insisting that aesthetic
appreciation (and by implication aesthetic creativity) is
closely involved with the basic laws of perception, but it
is going too far to say that aesthetic appreciation is completely reducible to these laws; this would ignore the
active striving and relational thinking which does at any
rate very frequently go with aesthetic satisfaction. If it is
true there is a general component in all varieties of
aesthetic appreciation, its presence in low degree may
account for the lack of artistic creativity in some able
individuals well able to draw. Conclusive evidence on
such matters cannot, however, be obtained from intercorrelational analysis, as the long and unresolved con-
troversy about the existence of a general factor in intelligence clearly indicates; only neurophysiological experimentation in conjunction with behavioural analysis can
settle these questions. The biological foundation of
Eysenck's law of aesthetic appreciation and its corollaries
is very insecure. It is entirely speculative and without
warrant in experimental neurophysiology to say that
nervous energy is decreased or drawn off in the manner
he suggests during perception, simple or aesthetic, nor is

there any evidence that changes of energy are related to feelings of pleasure in so simple a fashion. Furthermore, "nervous energy" in connection with aesthetic enjoyment has never been estimated chemically and biologists have merely been able to note increased blood flow when a group of nerve cells are particularly active. Creative and aesthetic activity requires a wide distribution of nerve-cell activity, and no measurements have been attempted yet. Electro-physiologically, V. J. and W. G. Walter recently (1949) made some interesting observations on the interrelation of mental and emotional changes and electro-encephalographic recording. They found that after a variety of photic stimulations, mental and emotional changes can be induced together with subjective visual sensations as indicated in E.E.G. records. They speculate that with appropriate psychological analysis some correlation could be found between E.E.G. features, the evoked responses and some such character as originality or creative imagination. But, rightly, they emphasize the speculative nature of this conclusion, and put the emphasis on the interrelations. So this pioneer work in the study of electro-physiologic expression of discrete mental mechanisms is far from offering a tool by which the "nervous energy" which Eysenck postulates may be measured quantitatively.

From the sociological point of view it is noteworthy that Eysenck ignores the relativity of aesthetic appreciation to cultural conditions in space and time. The history of art makes it clear that culturally acquired values have a complex interaction with simple unlearned preferences which rest on an innate physiological basis.

Nearly all experimental investigations into aesthetics have been concerned, like those of Eysenck, with appreciation rather than artistic expression and creativity. A notable exception is the work of C. Patrick (1933). She studied the creative process itself under standard conditions in 50 artists of some degree of eminence and in 50 non-artists by reading to them a poem and asking them to paint what it suggested to them, subsequently obtaining their introspections. She had previously compared the creative process in poets and non-poets by showing them a painting and asking them to write a poem suggested by it. Patrick described the psychological phases of the creative process in the terminology introduced by Graham Wallas: Preparation, Incubation, Illumination, Verification (or Revision). She modified his concept of incubation, however, by establishing that the incubated idea or mood is not entirely absent from awareness during that phase but recurs intermittently. Patrick's work confirms the essential importance of cognitive processes in aesthetic creativity. Her central finding was that the cognitive method of working was the same in all four groups, artists and non-artists, poets and non-poets. The trained individuals differed from the untrained in the effectiveness of their product, not in their manner of creating it. There were no cognitive differences in mode of work between artists and poets (they were, of course, carrying out different tasks), but certain conative differences impinged upon their working; the artists were better disciplined and more systematic owing to their formal training and were more inclined to seek the opinion of others owing to their more sociable mode of life. Patrick noted some differences in manner of intellectual approach within her groups but as her purpose was primarily to investigate general laws she did not pursue these.

That a thorough empirical investigation of pictorial art must deal both with aesthetic appreciation and with aesthetic expression or production is sufficiently plain. Such an investigation must consider both questions of neurophysiology and questions of sociology or cultural anthropology. Aesthetic preferences that depend on acquired training or cultural conditioning must be distinguished by careful experimentation from preferences that are characteristic of all human beings, irrespective of their training and background. The diffusion and interrelationships of the preferences dependent upon training and culture must be traced, and the neurophysiological basis of the universal preferences must be discovered. The differences in cognitive attitude and approach, such as Spearman's distinction of differences in breadth, must be analysed and their relationships and variations investigated. Such an ambitious programme would occupy several years, even taking into account the sporadic previous work done in the field of aesthetic appreciation. I cannot pretend in this study to be contributing substantially to this programme. But I wish to describe one difference of cognitive attitude which I believe to exist between pictorial artists and non-artists of equivalent intellectual ability, although I am aware that it needs empirical verification.

It is my belief that the relations in terms of which creative pictorial artists think tend much more to be those of situational conjunction * and much less those of classification than is the case with non-artists. I have been led to this view by clinical observations of the thinking processes in creative artists. It has also been suggested to me by the fact that pictorial activity is more prevalent among children and primitive peoples than among the ordinary adults in our society and that in those same groups thinking tends to be in terms of situational conjunction rather than classification. The enhanced pictorial activity of schizophrenic patients seems to me to depend in part on a shift of emphasis from classification to situational thinking. I do not intend by this to imply that the thinking of creative artists is abnormal; in the first place, I regard situational thinking as an entirely normal process, and secondly, in creative artists it is a question not of inability to think in classificatory terms, but merely of a preference for thinking situationally. The phenomena of dreams also suggest this possibility; dreams may be regarded as a sort of pictorial activity with certain obvious resemblances to painting and in dreams situa-

* By situational conjunction I mean relating objects according to their association in space or time as opposed to classifying them by the abstraction of common components. The difference between the two modes of thinking emerges with especial clarity on sorting tests, but is generally applicable.

tional thinking predominates over classificatory thinking. Recently the magazine *Picture Post* published an account by seven modern artists of their reasons for painting. There were certain differences in formulation but all said substantially the same thing. It was evident that all viewed their activity in painting as essentially relational, a task of discovering and expressing formal relationships in design. It was equally evident that their tendency was to think in terms of situational rather than classificatory relationships.

My hypothesis that pictorial artists tend to think situationally rather than in terms of classification has obvious affinities to the theory of K. Goldstein on abstract and concrete behaviour. On the basis of his work with brain-injured patients during and after the First World War and of more recent work by himself and his followers with brain-diseased, schizophrenic and oligophrenic patients, Goldstein distinguishes two fundamental capacity levels of the total personality, two modes of behaviour which he calls the abstract and the concrete attitudes. The normal person is capable of assuming both, whereas the abnormal individual tends to be confined to the concrete attitude. The concrete attitude is realistic, immediate and un-reflecting. The abstract attitude embraces more than merely the "real" stimulus in its scope; it implies conscious activity in the sense of reasoning, awareness and self-account of one's doing. The abstract attitude is marked by the presence and the concrete attitude by the absence of eight capacities. These are: (1) To detach our ego from the outer world or from inner experiences; (2) to assume a mental "set"; * (3) to account for acts to oneself and to verbalize the account; (4) to shift reflectively from one aspect of the situation to another; (5) to hold in mind simultaneously various aspects; (6) to grasp the essential of a given whole, to break up a given whole into parts, to isolate and to synthesize them; (7) to abstract common properties reflectively and to form hierarchic

* By "set" I mean a temporary condition of the organism which facilitates a certain specific type of activity.

concepts; (8) to plan ideationally, to assume an attitude towards the "more possible", and to think or perform symbolically.

Goldstein notes that normal individuals differ both in the ease with which they can adopt the abstract attitude and in their preference for doing so. He strongly maintains that there is a pronounced line of demarcation between the two attitudes which does not represent a gradual ascent from more simple to more complex mental sets. The abstract attitude demands the behaviour of a new energent quality, generically different from the concrete. From the evolutionary point of view this behavioural quality represents a recent achievement, a new functional level connected with the intact working of the cerebral cortex, especially the frontal lobes.

I am well aware of the damaging criticism to which Goldstein's theory has been subjected by many psychologists. J. McV. Hunt and others have pointed out that Goldstein's emphasis on the intensive study of individual cases and passionate rejection of statistical validation imports many sources of error and leads to a gross overgeneralization. Halstead, following Forster and von Monakow, observes that the brain-injured patients of the First World War were unsatisfactory material for investigating the problems which Goldstein poses. N. Cameron argues that Goldstein's eight criteria of the abstract are merely those customarily employed in demonstrating the intervention of consciousness and have no more valid application than in normal behaviour. Most psychologists feel that Goldstein paid inadequate attention to the intelligence level of his patients before the brain lesion; he ignores the approximately Gaussian distribution of intelligence and seems oblivious to the cognitive characteristics of dull normal and low average individuals. He also ignores the interaction with concrete and abstract thinking of special abilities and disabilities in dealing with verbal, spatial and mechanical relations. The most important criticism, however, is that of Hunt and Cameron, with which nearly all psychologists would agree; there is good reason to doubt the usefulness and validity of an effort to maintain separate categories of abstract and concrete behaviour, which seems to be a heritage of the Cartesian dichotomy between human and animal thinking. The assertion that abstract and concrete thinking are not acquired mental sets but fundamental capacity levels is more than dubious. Both require high levels of fundamental capacity, but neither arises automatically by maturation; both represent a complex accumulation of habits successively acquired.

If one cannot, however, accept without question Goldstein's assertion that abstract and concrete thinking represent fundamental capacity levels of the organism, one can agree that many aspects of abstract thinking are impaired in the brain-injured and also that normal individuals differ, probably to some extent independently of general intelligence, in the ease with which they think abstractly and in their preference for doing so.

Whether situational or categorical, the cognitive aspect seems a dominant factor in art. To-day's artists consciously analyse the total system of relations. This analysis has led them invariably to employ techniques which led to similarities between the schizophrenic and their own art products. In content the surrealists have explored "the subconscious" instead of external reality; schizophrenics reproduce their hallucinations and the world of their own. The cubists have analysed reality in terms of geometric interrelations; schizophrenics show a tendency for geometric ornamentation in the course of their disease. Chagall painted a man walking in the clouds, depicting an exalted feeling, and so experimented with the meaning of symbols; in schizophrenics the symbol becomes identical with the meaning and is reproduced as such. This experimentation of the moderns with form and content is naturally based to a greater extent on conscious intellectual activity than was, for instance, the work of the Renaissance artists. The emphasis is on conscious analysis which in its turn always makes the components more obvious, so that modern art products appear to present some degree of fragmentation. It was shown previously that in schizophrenics the basic disintegration is cognitive, leading also to fragmentation. Hence, the apparent similarities between modern and schizophrenic art.

VI

AN ILLUSTRATIVE CASE

I

WE HAVE DISCUSSED how far structural alterations in the brain and their subsequent functional manifestations in such activities as art, are related to one another. I have mentioned that the operation of leucotomy induces a bilateral and more or less symmetrical injury to the prefrontal lobes of the brain, and that after leucotomy, or, for that matter, closed head injuries, executive skill becomes altered, and the criteria of creativeness, so various authors have claimed, become altered as well. Whereas the observation that brain injury alters executive skill is fairly well established and has been demonstrated psychometrically, its results have not been studied in creative artists. Furthermore, observations in linking artistic creativeness and leucotomy still need to be verified: the investigations hitherto published concern a poet and not a painter.

As this study was being written a unique opportunity occurred: a creative artist was undergoing prefrontal leucotomy. The problems presented by such a case are these: first, does executive skill alter as it alters in non-artists; and secondly, does creative capacity alter? This was all the more suitable a case for special investigation because the illness of the patient altered the style of her pictorial expression. So a third problem is involved: an improvement of the psychosis raises the possibility of a renewed alteration in the patient's artistic style, which might be related to functional and structural changes.

The account given below is a synthesis based on the reports of the psychiatrist in charge of the case and on special psychological investigations.

Only a brief account of the patient's history can be given, to avoid any possibility of recognition; for the same reason, none of her drawings or paintings can be reproduced here.

The patient was an only child. There was a history of mental illness in her family on her mother's side. She was a normal baby, had a happy childhood and uneventful early schooldays. Her talent for painting very soon became apparent, and with the encouragement of teachers and artists who saw her work, she began a career as an artist. Her personality, however, altered at the onset of puberty; she became self-absorbed and moody. At the art school changes in her personality progressed till she broke down completely. She suffered from auditory hallucinations; the imaginary voices told her to commit suicide and she felt unable to resist. She was admitted to a psychiatric institute as an impulsive and suicidal patient.

In hospital, she received up-to-date physical methods of treatment and she improved slowly. She started painting again, but her work remained very restricted and academic. She could not express herself freely in painting because she felt she had to keep strictly to concrete objects in order to remain sane; abstract painting reminded her of the onset of her illness.

After discharge, she started life anew, went to a celebrated art school, but kept in close contact with her psychiatrist. About six months after her discharge, however, she relapsed again, heard imaginary voices, expressed delusions of persecution and became suicidal. She agreed to come back to the hospital; now she no longer cared what happened to her because she felt she could no longer paint.

After re-admission, she failed to respond to the normal

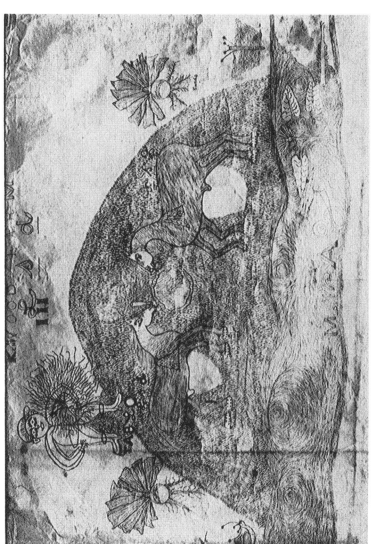

Fig. 13. 'Horses And Flooding'

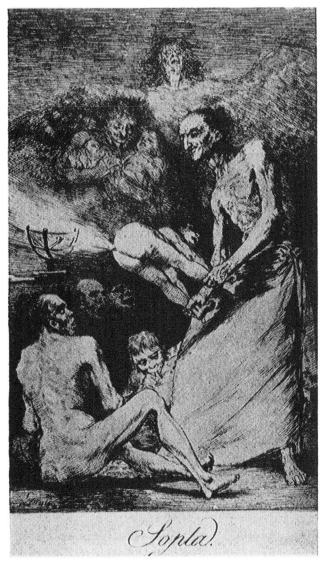

Fig. 14. Goya: Sopla

therapeutic procedures, so at last, with her consent, it was decided to perform an operation of leucotomy on her brain; the so-called lower quadrants of the prefrontal lobes were sectioned with a blunt instrument, according to the method described by W. Freeman. There were no complications, and the patient had an uneventful convalescence. Three weeks after the operation, she was more cheerful and communicative, and she worked almost daily on some picture. Her attitude towards her psychotic symptoms was fairly objective; she observed that they were present, but that they appeared somewhat diminished in intensity. She took an interest in her appearance, began to go out to visit her home, and made friendly contact with her parents and with her fellow patients. She was delighted to find that her creative capacity remained intact. At the time of writing (five weeks after the operation) she continues to make satisfactory progress as far as her personality is concerned.

As to the psychometric assessment of her case, after she was first admitted to hospital she was not in a suitable state for testing until several weeks had gone by. When it was judged that she was at last able to co-operate fruitfully in a psychometric investigation, she was tested with the Rorschach Ink Blots and also with Word-Association Responses. She was still vague, preoccupied and detached from her immediate environment. All the same, she grasped the nature of the Rorschach task immediately and settled down to it quite happily, perhaps because she was prepared for it by hearing other patients discuss it or perhaps because of her strong visual-mindedness. There was considerable difficulty in getting her to grasp the nature of the Word-Association task, either because she was unprepared for it or because of its verbal character.

Her treatment of the Ink Blots showed many distinctive features, schizophrenic in quality and especially interesting in one who was an artist. The forms she perceived were for the most part not clearly outlined, and were poorly integrated into meaningful structures. There was a curious disturbance in her perception of space relations

9

and relations of bodily parts. Thus in one blot she perceived a moth with its body, nose, wings and antennae distributed over the card in a quite unnatural way. In another she saw a volcano, presented in spatially incongruous sections; in still another she perceived a series of pelvises of increasingly poor form and constructed in a way suggestive of disordered spatial relations. She was incapable of any three-dimensional perceptions, which was unusual in an artist, and movement was almost completely absent in the forms she apprehended. She responded strongly to colour in the blots, but could not integrate the colours into meaningful shapes; thus she gave several pure colour responses, a schizophrenic reaction especially noteworthy in an artist. She made much use of black as a colour, an exceptional behaviour, which is generally a sign of affective disturbance. The content of her perceptions displayed little creativity; most of them were maps or anatomical representations; none were human beings. When she saw a map she was often confused and uncertain whether it was a real object she perceived or merely a conventional sign; thus in what she described as a map of Ireland she perceived at the same time pictures of real lakes and trees. When the matter was pursued, she declared that they were only conventional signs for lakes and trees, but her reaction suggested a disordered visual perception of her environment. Throughout her performance she tended to think in visualistic rather than conceptual terms. Her control over her reactions was considerably impaired, but she retained some degree of control.

She was asked to write her responses to the Word-Association test. They chiefly consisted of one word, empty of imaginative or emotional content. She appeared to be helpless when not confronted with matter which was concrete and presented visually. There were some odd defects in her reading and spelling. She showed considerable affective disturbance at the words "Mother" and "Father". The word "mother" led to a curious motor expression of this disturbance: she wrote "Mummy" with a proliferation of m's—Mummmmy. Some of her responses were suggestive of body-image disorder, for example: Month, *space*; Stomach, *small intestine*; organ, *lives*.

In both tests she gave the impression of an evasive, withdrawn personality, apparently lacking inner richness; she did not at this time express any paranoid feelings of suspicion or being wronged, nor did she indicate that apparently environmental events were specially significant for her.

After she had undergone treatment and just before she was discharged from hospital she was re-examined with the same tests. She had, according to her own account, no recollection of the previous testing. Her manner was still vague, but she was less preoccupied; her social behaviour was superficially more pleasant and she expressed greater interest in the tests. Her performance showed a considerably increased degree of control, but was no richer, no more imaginative. Her perceptions on the Rorschach Ink Blots were all reasonably good in form, clear in outline and meaningfully integrated. There was no evidence of a disturbance in spatial perceptions; although suggestions of disordered body imagery remained. Three-dimensional perceptions, movement and human figures appeared this time. There were many fewer maps and anatomical responses; concrete, inanimate objects and animals took their place. Her colour reactivity was less marked, less schizophrenic in quality, more controlled; the colour percepts were all organized into meaningful shapes. This time she made no use of black as a colour. In the Word-Association test she showed no affective disturbances. Her responses consisted of several words, but they were all definitions without imaginative or emotional content. She expressed no attitudes of being wronged nor did her manner show any suspicion or distrust. In comparison with her previous performance, both tests indicated that she had adjusted herself superficially and had mastered for the time being an underlying schizophrenic reactivity.

After she returned to hospital she was tested with the

Behn Ink Blots, a series parallel to the Rorschach Ink Blots. She was also tested with these again under the influence of methedrine. In comparison with her earlier performances, what was most marked on both occasions was the emergence of suspicions, of distrustful behaviour and the expression of feelings that she had been wronged and ill-treated. She believed also that events had special reference to herself. This corresponded to changes which had been observed in her clinically. There were several other differences. Her reactivity to colour was much less marked and she showed some tendency to avoid it. She made use of the white spaces in the ink-blots to construct percepts, a behaviour entirely absent in her earlier performances; this is usually interpreted as a sign of opposition, contrary reaction or negativism. Queer forms of verbalization, a trend only hinted at in the previous testing, appeared explicitly. Thus she modified her description of a cat she had perceived to: *It's rather the desire to wanting to catch a bird*. When the Word-Association test was re-administered to her, such verbalizations were several times evident; examples are: Disease, *Something, germ, that makes your health ill*; and Kiss: *Mouth to mouth and face to face—a conveyance of thought and love*. Her Word-Association responses once more were chiefly definitions, but they had now a distinct emotional component in them, an expression of paranoid or wronged feeling.

When she was tested with the Behn Ink Blots under the influence of methedrine, some of these trends disappeared, others were more explicitly revealed. There were no odd verbalizations, and she organized the different parts of the blots into more competent and imaginative percepts than she had ever done previously. She avoided colour in a more marked degree; there was an increase in her perceptions of movement and a marked increase in her use of white spaces. Another interesting change was the emergence of a content in her responses which was menacing or provocative of fear; for example, what she perceived originally as a barn-owl, became under the influence of methedrine "a terrifying winged skull".

Probably this content had previously been suppressed rather than not experienced. Body-image disturbance was not apparent in these performances.

After leucotomy she was once more tested with the Rorschach Ink Blots. Her manner at the beginning was still distrustful and full of suspicion, but afterwards she relaxed and became more co-operative. The disturbance in spatial perception, shown in her very first performance, was again evident, but not in so clear-cut a form. There was also a renewed suggestion of disordered body-imagery; the injury to her head appeared to be a component in this disturbance. Avoidance of colour-responses was more marked than ever before; she openly expressed her dislike of the colours. In her sparing use of them she was much affected emotionally, as if they represented a potential danger to her. The outline, structuring and organization of her responses were poorer than at any time except in the first performance of all. There were again some queer verbalizations.

The general impression of her final performance was that her fundamental schizophrenic reactivity was unaltered, but that her concern, self-criticism and control were diminished. The suggestion was that her contact with her human environment was improved.

II

Her paintings before her illness had shown great originality, an imaginative perceptual treatment and courageous handling of colours and of structural relations. She had inclined towards ornamentation and strongly marked patterning; by choice, her paintings had always been of small size. Whilst her illness developed, her drawings were not altered by her early psychotic experiences; the first influence of which occurred the night before she came into the hospital. She had been working during the afternoon on a design of two horses, grazing: black horses on a green background, executed in green and black Indian ink. In the night she suddenly jumped out of bed, took a pen and, apparently under the influence of auditory hallucinations, felt compelled to finish the drawing. She drew five shields in the background, with a different crest on each of them. These have no meaning and are not originally connected with the picture; superficially they might be looked upon as expressions of bizarre reactivity. Her own account of this drawing, of the adding of symbols to "real things", has been mentioned in her case history above. Whilst in hospital and under treatment she did not paint. Between her discharge and re-admission, when her psychosis became active again, she reproduced her hallucinatory experiences. At that time she worked with pencil only. After she was re-admitted she could not work at all. She was given methedrine injections and while the action of this sympathetico-mimetic drug lasted, she worked in un-inhibited fashion; but as soon as the effect of the drug wore off, she relapsed into her self-absorbed, depressed and hallucinatory state. The four pictures she painted under methedrine were: "The Tiger, from the Tiger's Point of View", "A Washstand and a Bed", "A Chair" and "A Cart". All were of large size, were disproportionate to the space, and were drawn—studies in sepia and white —with very heavy contours; they retained artistic value. Then came the operation. Before this she had just begun to outline a horse; six days after her operation she began to paint again. Once more she used monochrome tech-nique and drew the outline of a nude. The picture was completely out of proportion to the space provided; she worked happily on it, but did not like anyone to see it. One day she asked for vinegar, to make the flesh of the nude more human (*sic!*), then suddenly she tore it up. When I asked her about her painting, she said that she could use her old technique now, but she did not want to do so. At present she is interested only in the actual relation of shapes, which is "reality". She is no longer afraid of non-reality, but is not interested in it. She tore up her nude because it was not what she wanted, and she had no more use for it. Apparently her painting was an experience of her own and not intended to afford aesthetic satisfaction to others. In her third post-operative week she remembered that before the operation she had begun to draw a horse; she said that she knew exactly what she wanted to do about it, and wanted to work on it again. Once more the picture started as a monochrome, though now and then she put white patches on the sepia. Again the spatial relations were out of proportion. The horse occupied the whole of the paper, so she pinned another piece of paper to it, and painted a cart behind the horse. A week later she added another piece of paper to the picture and drew a man standing in the cart. Thus the picture became L-shaped. Whilst working she wished that she had a very large canvas because she wanted to do paintings that were greater than life-size.

To investigate changes in her executive skill induced by the operation special tests were administered to her three days before the operation; the same tests were repeated at three and at twenty-four days after the operation. The tests used were mainly based on the perception, analysis and reproduction of spatial relations. Besides these the Reitman Pin-Man test was applied on each occasion. The spatial tests consisted of Kohs' Blocks, the Bender Visual-Motor Gestalt test, and four tests of drawing ability adapted from Clark L. Hull—Memory for Designs, Circle Completion, Angle Copying and Size Copying. It has been established that after leucotomy patients tend to show an impaired performance on the first two of these spatial tests. The last four tests were included among those employed by Hull in investigating the ability to execute freehand drawing; he did not find them all of utility in this matter but to my particular purpose they seemed relevant. In the Kohs' test the subject is given cubes coloured differently on each side and is required to construct patterns with them in imitation of patterns shown to him on cards; as the test proceeds, the number of blocks and the complexity of the patterns are both increased. The Bender test is widely recognized as a delicate indicator of impaired capacity owing to organic cerebral damage. It presents to the subject a number of rather unusual designs, deriving from the Gestalt figures of Wertheiner, and requires him either to copy them or to reproduce them from memory; in this case reproduction from memory was required. Hull's Memory for Designs resembles the Bender test, but the figures are somewhat easier to remember and reproduce. In the Circle Completion test, the subject is given arcs of circles and required to complete them by freehand drawing; in Angle Copying he has to reproduce various angles as closely as possible; in Size Copying he is shown a square, a circle, a triangle and a Latin cross and required to copy each so that it is as near in size to the original as possible.

Before the operation the patient's performance on all these tests was highly competent. Contrary to expectation little or no impairment was evident three days after the operation. On the twenty-fourth day, however, changes were more apparent. She found it more difficult to analyse some of the Kohs' Block designs. The Bender figures were much less satisfactorily reproduced; there were reversals of direction and displacements of parts, simplifications of the design, changes in length and relative size, flattening of curves and similar changes. None of these features appeared in her two previous testings. The lines were notably thicker than before. Another important change was that on the first two occasions the separate figures were systematically and effectively arranged on the page; on the third occasion they were scattered over the page haphazardly and ineffectively. The Memory for Designs test showed on the third occasion simplification of the figures, increase in size and thicker lines; on the first two occasions the reproduction was all but perfect. Neither in the Bender test nor in Memory for Designs did she show any change in purely motor execution; the change was in the spatial relations of the design. The Circle Completion test showed no change even at the third testing, except for some thickening of the lines. In the Angle Copying test the reproductions were increased in size and thickness on the twenty-fourth day. So far as Size Copying was concerned, the reproductions were always exceedingly close but they were more exact on the first two occasions; there was a slight tendency to increase of size the third time. In the Pin-man test the verbal responses were substantially the same on all three occasions. The Pin-man drawing, however, showed some changes. On the first and second occasions it was exceedingly good, worthy of an artist. On the third occasion the drawing was mediocre; it would have been passable in a non-artist, but was well below the level of an artist. There was a perceptible weakening in the suggestive character of the figure. In particular the arms were poorly drawn; they were mere empty copying. Besides this, the figure was disposed in the available space very ineffectively; it was displaced into a corner of the sheet. This would have meant nothing in a non-artist, but was significant in a patient of high aesthetic ability in pictorial art.

Only a few conclusions can be drawn with any degree of certainty from her immediate post-operative condition. The style, which had begun to alter just before the operation, continued to alter in a more marked way. The pre-operative alteration of her style was ascertainable only under the influence of methedrine. So far as I have been able to observe, the paintings of patients under the influence of methedrine show a marked fragmentation, whereas her pictures under the drug were large and well-balanced structures. Thus it may be that the methedrine treatment did no more than mobilize her new style which was maintained by the post-operative personality. In this sense, the alteration of her style has probably little to do with the operation.

She did not lose her executive skill, a fact also evidenced by the Bender test. This might be expected, in that an artist's executive skill is such an established behaviour that relatively restricted damage to the prefrontal lobes might leave it unaltered. It should, however, be recalled that neurological observations suggest that after cerebral damage the loss of skills precedes the loss of more elementary functions.

On the other hand, the changes registered by the Bender test confirmed that there were alterations in her treatment of spatial relations, just as her drawings had indicated. This might quite easily be a sequel to her brain injury, but other explanations are possible. It may well be that her perception of space was altered as a result of the operation. The post-operative responses to the Rorschach test might be taken to support this explanation.

Another interpretation of this fact might be based on post-operative changes in personality, the existence of which is widely recognized. An artist must have a pre-liminary concept of the structural relations he is going to paint; the concept and the canvas together shape the unity of the finished work. In her case, it seems that the preliminary schema is somehow only vaguely organized and remains fluid, so that the canvas has to be addition-ally enlarged according to changes in her visual con-ception. Now, as I have already noted, it is said that after leucotomy the ultimate evaluation of planned action, or foresight in general, becomes affected. Thus it may be that what is expressed in her bad structural unity is a disturbed capacity for planning, which leads to an un-satisfactory manifestation of spatial relations. The evalua-tion of planned action, or "foresight", however, is a complex activity comprising several components, one of which is motivation. Assuming her psychosis to be included among the motivating forces, one can state that her motivations did alter, as judged by favourable changes as far as her behaviour in the hospital was concerned and also in her activities outside the hospital. On the other hand, this hardly explains the alterations in spatial per-ception. Furthermore, A. F. Tredgold has described a mental defective who was cared for during a period of many years in an institution and who showed a highly developed capacity for planning, as evidenced by the construction of model ships, some of which were exhibited with great success. After this patient's death, the examina-tion of the brain demonstrated, amongst other anomalies, badly underdeveloped prefrontal and temporal lobes.

Thus structural deficiencies in the cortex and artistic foresight do not seem to be in close correlation with one another.

Apart from the fact that the patient's pictorial expression altered, the conclusions to be drawn are tentative and none gives a direct answer to the problems which were raised in the introduction. The study of one case cannot offer a secure basis for generalization on such matters, for instance, as whether leucotomy is likely to influence artistic production favourably or unfavourably. It certainly affects non-artists differently, as I indicated in the previous chapter. To a certain degree it is entirely specific to the individual how much of the prefrontal lobes can be damaged without causing marked deficit in the patient's artistic capacity. All one can state is that the study of one artist showed that a special cerebral injury caused alteration in the personality, but affected creation only superficially and not fundamentally up to the beginning of the fifth post-operative week. A more decisive answer could be given only if such a case were followed up and studied over a period of three or four years.

VII

INTERPRETATION OF
PSYCHOTIC ART

Sublimation and the functional significance of art (Freud)—Criticism of the psycho-analytical approach—Jung's concept of symbols and criticism of it—Typology, another aspect of the motivation of art—Application of the interpretative approaches in the pathographies—Pathographic sketch of Goya—Problems arising from pathographies.

I

WE HAVE NOW examined the manner in which the psychotic picture has been regarded in its form or its content as symptomatic of a special illness, and we have discussed attempts to relate form and content to the dynamics of the patient's illness, that is to say, to the basic motivations and needs on which his illness depends and to his particular way of responding to such fundamental drives. Dynamic views in relation to psychotic art led to interpretative speculations on the motivation of art products in general and also in the case of individual artists. These interpretative attempts should now be more closely scrutinized.

The first attempt to solve the problems of art by an interpretation in dynamic terms was the contribution of Freud to the understanding of aesthetic creativity. Freud first posed the question, What function has creativity for the artist himself? In his study of Leonardo da Vinci and elsewhere he demonstrated the symbolic expression in the artist's works of subconscious conflicts. Put in another way, he introduced the notion of the subconscious as a motivating force in creative activity. At the same time he argued about the cathartic function of art. This last concept was presented in especially clear form by Baudouin, who maintained that art represents a relief from tension and that as such it can be a therapeutic agent in nervous diseases. Release from tension by means of creativity is an application of the well-known psychoanalytical concept of sublimation which is regarded as a symbolic expression of subconscious conflicts. For the pictorial artist the symbols are non-verbal substitutes for something meaningful. The function of the symbol is equated to the role of symbols in dreams; that is to say, it conceals the real meaning from the artist as from the dreamer, and it graduates and reduces emotions which in direct, non-symbolic expression would arouse disturbance, stress or extreme unhappiness. In non-symbolic expression such emotions would be chaotic: they would not be co-ordinated. By reducing their objects to symbolic form the emotions are rendered orderly and tolerable. This process of symbol formation is one of Freud's well-known mechanisms, together with displacement and condensation, the function of which in psychotic art I have already discussed.

In this approach the interpretation of the symbols is entirely based on Freud's theory of the *libido*. It is assumed that the fundamental conflicts of the artist and the notions most disturbing to him must necessarily lie in the sexual sphere. The fact that in many instances there are more urgent and immediate sources of conflict is disregarded. The psycho-analytic investigators describe a legion of phallic symbols. There is no independent evidence that the majority of these are in fact symbols for the male organ. A similar criticism applies to the other Freudian symbols. In the case of one individual it may sometimes be satisfactorily demonstrated that a particular object symbolizes a given meaning. To extend this fact to an assertion that the object symbolizes the same meaning for all other individuals is quite unwarrantable. Nevertheless it has been a common procedure among psycho-analytic investigators. It may also be noted that in symbolic interpretations along these lines there is marked disagreement between one psycho-analyst and another about the meaning to be attached to a given symbol in an art product. The subjectivity of this approach condemns it as a scientific method of attack.

The concept of the functional significance of art for the psychotic artist has been further elaborated by Kris, who has argued that the art of psychotics is a means of adjustment to reality. Other psycho-analysts have demonstrated in specific instances that the choice of theme in art is dependent on conflicts within the artist. These studies have succeeded in showing that the motivations leading to the production of art by the artist may be highly significant in his life-history. They have also shown (see Chapter 8) that such motivations may correspond to general needs and drives in the community; it is upon this fact that appreciation and enjoyment of art by the general public depends, at any rate, in part. These accounts in terms of motivation, however, fail to give a satisfactory description and evaluation of art as a function of the human organism specific to it.

Another psycho-analytic explanation of the phenomenon of art, only seemingly different from the one just considered, is that it is closely allied to play. The slow maturation of the human infant makes it necessary that the parents should provide protection for it and satisfaction for its oral needs. The child, identifying himself with his parents, engages in mock activities of protection and the provision of oral satisfaction. These activities give him pleasure and constitute what is ordinarily called play. Because play has a pleasure value it helps the child to tolerate the difficulties and frustrations of things as they are, called by Freud "the reality principle". By means of play the child learns to postpone satisfactions, a capability essential to ordered social life. At a later stage of cultural development the play of the child evolves into rituals and art with an accompanying process of rationalization. It will be evident that this explanation overlooks many aspects both of play and of art. In particular it neglects the conceptual qualities of art, which I have already considered. The theory of the evolution of art from play will be seen to rest on the Freudian pleasure-principle and ultimately on the theory of sexual *libido*. It is, therefore, vulnerable to all the criticism directed against these hypotheses.

Clearly the psycho-analytical evaluation of art is closely interwoven with Freudian doctrines in general. It could hardly be otherwise. For this reason we must re-state, as briefly as possible, the objections to the Freudian theories from the standpoint of general scientific knowledge. In a grossly over-simplified manner, psycho-analysis treats psychological processes and reactions as causally determined. Human behaviour is linked up into a rigid system of cause and effect with a concept of cause which is not only fallaciously narrow but is for the most part purely hypothetical. One might mention here the interesting contradiction, noted by K. Young, that the technical tool of so ultra-deterministic a system of psychology is "free association". In relating each item of human behaviour to an over-simplified determinant or system of determinants psycho-analysis ignores the great differences in the strength of the motivating drives leading to people's actions and the enormous variation that exists in the meaningfulness of actions to the individual. Thus a patient's delusions that his testes are being snipped off by an hallucinatory pair of scissors and some individual's habit of pulling leaves from trees are treated on the same level as consequences of a castration complex. The Freudian psychology neglects the fact that large numbers of human actions are merely habitual or, to use Goldstein's term, "preferred" positions or modes of response, having no meaningful relation to the individual's basic motivating drives. So far as the fundamental drives themselves are concerned, by centring all attention on reproductive behaviour psycho-analysis gives wholly insufficient weight to the importance for the organism of what E. S. Russell calls its "maintenance activities", its endeavour to preserve its integrity against its inanimate and animate environment, its behaviour in relation to nutrition and to enemies and the like. Rather similarly by centring attention on the affective aspect of human psychological deficiencies and disabilities the psycho-analytic approach underrates the importance of purely cognitive factors, resting on neural structure and function, in such inadequacies; this is especially shown in the Freudian treatment of the phenomena of memory, difficulties in remembering names or facts, slips of the tongue or pen, and such matters.

From a biological point of view the Freudian theory is one-sided. Considered sociologically its weaknesses are even more striking. Freud based his system of psychology on his theory of the development of personality. The child begins as a polymorph pervert. Then it becomes sexually attracted to the mother; an accompanying sexual jealousy of the father leads in the male child to the formation of the Oedipus complex. The succession of events in the female child is more complicated and obscure. From the moment that the mother-fixation and the Oedipus complex are formed the whole structure becomes one of accumulated complexes. This leads almost naturally to the conclusion of Roheim that civilization and culture are basically pathological in nature; they are a compensatory reaction to infantile conflicts. Here it must be observed that there is no satisfactory proof of the existence of the Oedipus situation. On the contrary the careful investigation of C. W. Valentine with the children of English professional workers suggests that it is a quite erroneous description of the true state of affairs. Field research in societies and cultures other than our own, notably the work of B. Malinowski and the anthropologists of the school of F. Boas, has shown the existence of systems of values and attitudes wholly incompatible with Freud's

hypothesis. It is unnecessary to stress the extreme im-
probability of Freud's theory that there was a primal
horde in which the dominating father was slain and that
the feelings of guilt aroused by this murder were the
starting-point of civilization; recent attempts to treat this
theory as untrue historically but true "endopsychically"
have made it no more plausible. Considered sociologically
and anthropologically the whole psycho-analytic theory
is deficient because it neglects the differential effects of
culture and the social environment on the child's development. It is true that in the majority of cases the most
influential persons in shaping the child's attitudes, values
and standards are its parents, especially its mother; but
those parents are themselves part of a more or less complex
social pattern in relation to which the values that they
instil into the child vary in nature or emphasis. Besides
this, the individual's personality and strivings cannot be
said to be rigidly determined in early infancy. The
human organism carries a number of inherited psychological tendencies, but it is especially characterized by
its plasticity of behaviour. This plasticity is greater
in childhood than later and becomes progressively less;
even so it remains throughout life, save in pathological cases. The plastic human organism from early
infancy onwards is in continual functional relationship
with a complex social structure; all the time it is
being modified in its strivings and its attitudes by that
relationship. The Freudian psychologists grossly over-
simplify this social structure and give little attention to its
importance.

The relevance of this criticism to psycho-analytical
interpretations of art products, pictorial and otherwise,
will be readily apparent. The great service of the psycho-
analysts in showing that art has a dynamic motivation
must be recognized; their over-simplified and one-sided
account of that motivation must be rejected. It should be
noted here that a Freudian formulation may at times be
found to give the most adequate description of a particular psychopathological case. The essential criticism

10

of the psycho-analysts is not that they state what is untrue in a particular individual but that they fallaciously extend into general laws what has been demonstrated only in a special instance. For further basic criticisms of Freud's teaching I would refer the reader to the works of Sturt, Wohlgemuth and Jastrow.

Systems of psychology which have developed out of psycho-analysis have taken their point of departure from a keen feeling of the shortcomings of the Freudian theory in one field or another of psychopathology. They have attempted to correct these shortcomings. Jung's revision of the psycho-analytical approach began on biological lines by endeavouring to broaden the narrow concept of the libido. This he did by calling all the strivings of the organism "libido" and by postulating a system of multiple and deepening psychological layers in the individual such as the "persona", the "anima", "the personal unconscious" and the "racial and collective unconscious". Jung found that in the course of analysis the symbols became universal and expressed collective images such as Good and Evil, instead of Mother and Father. He maintains that these symbols originate from that part of the unconscious which is primordial; furthermore, these symbols have never been conscious and never personal. They represent some kind of pre-thought, an experience partly emotional and partly cognitive, which has been handed down to the individual through generations from the dim past. These pre-thoughts or symbols cannot be verbalized; they can only be experienced as an urge for the universal, for the spiritual; they are the "creative urge". It is possible that phantasy will express those pre-thoughts in an adequate way. Hence the study of phantasy-products, such as the drawings of patients, can give direct access to the deepest layers of the personality and so the therapist is enabled to help the patient to achieve a moral balance.

These Jungian symbols are looked upon as the right and only way to express the universal, so naturally the "analytical", that is, the Jungian psychologists, have collected an immense wealth of paintings from psycho-neurotic and psychotic patients during the course of treatment. In the Jungian analysis, by means of painting the *mandala*, a symbol of concentric structure, makes its repeated appearance. This contrasts with the drawings obtained from their patients by non-Jungian psycho-therapists, in which the mandala does *not* appear. One of the best known works which thoroughly illustrates the Jungian approach is Baynes's *Mythology of the Soul*; I may note that the far-reaching conclusions reached by this author are based on the study of only two cases. Another example of recent works written under Jung's influence, which I choose at random, is M. Petrie's *Art and Regeneration* (1946). This author has attempted a comprehensive survey of art from a Jungian viewpoint, including the *mandalas* and all Jung's theoretical constructs. There is little originality in the formulae of her work, but it is a representative sample of the approach to art problems made by this school. The methodological freedom that she permits herself leaves small room for objectivity. "The existence of the unconscious is now regarded as an estab-lished fact", she writes; this would be more accurate scientifically if "working hypothesis" were substituted for "fact". The number of other art books, written in terms of the Jungian theory, is enormous. For the understanding of art, it would be less valuable to discuss all this literature than to discuss the general scientific objections to Jung's concepts.

It is highly questionable whether the Jungian symbols actually "express" collective images or whether they are merely so interpreted. The chief proof offered that they are such an expression is the introspective account of the patient; alternatively the Jungian interpretation itself may be presented as evidence. In either case the argument rests on entirely subjective grounds, and in the second eventuality is circular. The Jungian method of approach is *a priori* and not empirical. Furthermore, as Boas and his collaborators have repeatedly pointed out, anthropological evidence indicates the relativity of all symbols and the universality of none. Ruth Bunzel has fully demonstrated this relativity of symbols in a number of diverse cultural patterns. If it is shown empirically that there is no universality of symbols, then the central pillar of the Jungian system falls to the ground. Another objection to this symbolic theory is grounded in Jung's conception, already mentioned, that the symbols have never been conscious or personal and cannot be verbalized. If they cannot be verbalized then they cannot be apprehended rationally, and they are insusceptible of scientific treatment. The whole Jungian theory then becomes antithetical to a scientific approach. One must here remark that medical psychology, which is a branch of biology, cannot operate with valuative concepts such as "good" and "evil"; its sole value as a theoretical science is truth and as an applied science the adjustment of patients, and not their moral balance. The introduction of other values shifts psychology from the empirical sciences into the fold of metaphysical, ethical and normative inquiry. Nicole has already raised the question: Is Jung a scientist or is he a prophet?

Whilst certain paintings clearly suggest to the Jungian psychologist the rudiments of the *mandala*, the same paintings with equal clarity suggest phallic symbols to the psycho-analytical spectator. It seems probable that the contradictory interpretations depend on the projective processes of the onlooker; he sees what he expects or is predisposed to see. On the other hand, it is certainly a fact that pictures produced by patients do actually reflect in a clear manner the viewpoint of their particular therapist. There is nothing surprising about this. The analyst interprets the picture to the patient according to his own enlightenment. Thus he influences him in the production of the next one. So it proceeds. Ultimately the pictures are diagnostic only for the therapist's creed. Whether art is interpreted from one viewpoint or the other, each school offers merely a subjective basis for its estimation. The problem of art is fitted into a pre-existing theory; such fitting of problems to prior theories was a typical feature of continental psychological work in the early twentieth century.

Other investigators have inquired into the motivation of artistic creativity from a different standpoint. These workers, though their aims have varied, may be grouped as Typologists. It is difficult, when surveying this vast field of typology, to present it systematically, and only a few representative theories can be considered. Jaensch, whose work I have mentioned, extended his theory of eidetic imagery to artistic productions; he recognized different styles of work corresponding to his classification of types based on the presence or absence of eidetic phenomena, that is, corresponding to his tetanoid, basedowoid, epileptoid and other types. Lowenfeld, studying the artistic productions of blind artists, distinguished two types on another perceptual basis, a visual and a haptic type or type dependent on the sense of touch. Jung built up a quite different typology, not on the basis of perception but on that of fundamental attitude (introvert and extravert) modified by the four mental functions into which he analysed mind, namely, Thinking, Feeling, Intuition and Sensation. He applied this typology in evaluating art, a procedure pushed *ad absurdum* by Evans. Like the whole of Jung's system, this typology rests on prior and not empirical grounds. The basic attitudes of introversion and extraversion are not defined in precise and verifiable terms. They comprise a number of distinct psychological variables, such as degree of responsiveness to inner mental constructions rather than outer presentations, degree of introspectiveness and self-analysis, degree of emotional expressiveness, degree of sociability, degree of conformity to social norms, and other tendencies. Common observation and experimental studies, such as those of J. P. Guildford, alike indicate that the concomitant variation of such tendencies is never more than moderately high. Still more important, there is no break in their occurrence sharply dividing those individuals who show them from those who do not. On the contrary they are distributed, when any population is surveyed, in a graduated form from minimal to maximal incidence with the great majority of individuals showing a given tendency to more or less the same extent; their distribution usually approximates to a Gaussian curve. Moreover, in different situations an individual shows a given tendency to varying extents. The type concept distorts the facts. As for the four mental functions, it may be said that no psychologist outside the Jungian school accepts this analysis as either true or convenient. Most British, as opposed to American and Continental, psychologists still find it useful to distinguish the traditional three processes or aspects of human behaviour and experience, namely, Thinking, Feeling and Striving, but these processes are regarded as interlocked and always present in a psychological phenomenon in greater or less degree. One of these aspects may be more marked in a certain individual's behaviour than in the behaviour of others, but there is no warrant for believing that any individual operates chiefly by one process to the exclusion of the others. The Jungian analysis ignores the conative aspect, but adds the new functions of intuition and sensation. This addition is pointless; the processes called intuition and sensation can be satisfactorily described as special forms of thinking in conjunction with feeling. If one is to discriminate such special forms one could make a much larger number than four. The existence of types of individuals using one (or two) of these functions to the exclusion of the others has not been confirmed by empirical researches.

The introvert-extravert dichotomy of Jung is akin to that of Kretschmer, based upon structure of the body. Kretschmer's typology is the best known and most widely employed of all which rest on a distinction between constitutional characteristics. It may be regarded as fundamental to all subsequent work along those lines. Kretschmer calls constitution "the totality of inborn peculiarities"; all the affective and voluntary reaction of the individual he names character; and he applies the term temperament to the psychic tempo or the "tempo of performance". These terms have been employed with somewhat different meanings by other workers such as McDougall and Willemse. Kretschmer distinguishes four chief typical types, the pyknic, the asthenic or leptosomatic, the athletic and the dysplastic, and he finds that these are correlated to two main types of temperamental reaction, the cyclothymic and the schizothymic. The cyclothymes correspond to the pyknic physical type, the schizothymes to the other three types of constitution. The cyclothymes are in good harmony with their external environment, the schizothymes opposed to or detached from it. So far as artists are concerned he groups the realists and humorists with the cyclothymes, as for example Wilhelm Busch, and the "pathetics", romantics and formalists with the schizothymes, as for example Grünewald.

A number of investigators have found confirmation for Kretschmer's correlation of body-type to psychological characteristics; a number have not. There tends to be an increasing doubt of his thesis in its bare and simple form, though not of the basic proposition that somatic structure is a determinant of psychological and psychopathological reaction. The chief difficulty in his theory, as in the Jungian and all other typologies, is that the vast majority of individuals are mixed in type. It corresponds more closely to the facts to think not of types but of factors or components which exist in varying measure in each individual. Nearly all investigators have found a quite considerable number of cases in which the psychological reaction of the individual, healthy or morbid, is in contradiction to what would be expected from his somatic characteristics, if the Kretschmerian theory were true. This may be in part accounted for in terms of the varying mixture of components and in part due to the fact that experience, learning and the influence of the environment can transform the basic mode of psychological reaction. Kretschmer's anthropometric techniques leave much to be desired. Moreover, Eysenck has drawn attention to the dubious validity of many of the conclusions drawn from the measurements; for instance, among

Kretschmer's pathological cases, the differences found within the schizophrenic group are almost as great as the differences between that group and the group of manic-depressives. Sheldon has developed more exact anthropometric techniques than Kretschmer and has modified the over-simple notion of types into the more appropriate one of varying components, for which he has evolved an ingenious system of measurement. He has also endeavoured to correlate constitutional to psychological differences, but his work in the latter regard is less satisfactory than his anatomical results.

All these typological researches remain problematic but, again, like the efforts of the great psycho-pathological schools, they have led to attempts to interpret the motivation of artistic activity.

A practical application of these motivational approaches was found in the study of the life-histories of well-known artists. Such work became an attractive sideline of psychiatry; psychiatrists of various schools produced in abundance pathographic studies. The earlier workers have emphasized the psychopathological aspect only, but pathographers of later date put the emphasis on the art itself. Thus Schilder, when studying *Alice in Wonderland*, drew conclusions about the nature of nonsense poetry. Kris examined the nature of caricatures from a psycho-analytical viewpoint. Non-psychiatric biographies of morbid personalities have also helped to enrich our knowledge of psychotic art in relation to the artist. An example is *The Quest for Corvo*, Symon's study of F. Rolfe. The classical work on pathography, now somewhat outdated, is that of Lange and Eichbaum. They define pathography as a "demonstration of the markedly abnormal or pronouncedly morbid aspects of an historic and famous character". These two authors went far enough by not sparing anyone in their search for the pathological. To elucidate, however, what is aesthetically incomprehensible in an artist's production by correlating it to his psycho-neurotic illness is only possible if there is a positive correlation between his illness and his art. Weygandt has described two negative and two positive relationships that might subsist between mental illness and art. He suggests that illness might not affect art or it might extinguish art altogether; as a positive correlation he thinks that illness might facilitate a dormant talent or it might cause a change of style. It is this last possibility that has usually given a working hypothesis to pathographers in their examination of the art products of "morbid artists".

To demonstrate the pathographic technique it will be of value to make use of this approach in outlining a sketch of the life and works of a celebrated artist, who showed psycho-pathological features. The artist I shall examine is Goya.

II

Francisco Jose de Goya y Lucientes was born in 1746. His grandfather on his mother's side was mentally ill, but there is no further record of illness in his heredity. As a child he was brought up in the provinces; even there his talent aroused attention, and as early as 1759 he began to study in an art school in Zaragoza, where he remained for six years, during which time the awkward country boy developed into a pugnacious, gay young man. The few documents which refer to these school years are not entirely reliable, and it is a difficulty in making this study that very little of the evidence about Goya's life is reliable. Men were killed one night in a rowdy scuffle; apparently Goya was implicated, and according to some authors was suspected by the Inquisition; other writers attribute the Inquisition's interest to another affair. At all events, Goya fled and appeared in Madrid in 1765. He involved himself in amorous adventures; consequently his biographers consider it a matter of course that he should be found stabbed on one occasion. Some authors hold that it was not till this period that the Inquisition regarded Goya as a suspicious character; others maintain that information against him was laid with the police. Goya fled once more. He left Spain with a troupe of toreadors, and eventually arrived in Italy, alone, forsaken and with little money. It is in Italy that he is first referred to as an artist. His adventures multiplied in Rome, and he had to flee for the third time. The most diverse reasons are given for this, as, for example, that he was arrested when trying to abduct a girl from a convent and was freed only by the intervention of the Spanish ambassador, who thereupon sent him home. This is no more reliable than the story that he climbed the spire on the dome of St. Peter's.

Whatever the truth may be, Goya by 1771 had returned to Zaragoza, where he lived nearly two years in an abbey for which he was painting frescoes. In 1775 we again find him in Madrid. He was now a married man; his wife was Josefa Bayeau, sister to the court painter, whose earnings, by reason of his technical conservatism, were high. Goya's wife was extremely attached to her brother, and he played a large part in the family quarrels. The marriage was unhappy; suffering silently all the time from her husband's infidelity, his wife bore him twenty children and then died.

From 1775 Goya's position and income increased, and he received commissions from the Court. At this time he painted the cartoons for the carpets in the Prado. Delightful colours, charming compositions, attractive choice of theme characterize these genre pictures. The religious pictures he was commissioned to paint are likewise full of harmony. By 1780 he was a member of the Academy and was beginning to paint portraits, being by this time a man of wealth and consequence. In 1788 Charles IV ascended the Spanish throne. The king was weak, the queen ruled through her lovers, morality gradually disappeared from the court and corruption was rife. Goya was appointed court painter, and became acquainted with the Infanta Alba. His legendary relationship with her has been coloured by his biographers with many phantasies. For some time he lived in retirement, according to some biographers, with the Infanta; in this seclusion he began the peculiar series of engravings known as "Los Caprichos" (1793).

These were different from anything else he had produced. The engravings, according to their content, can be divided into several groups. Each has a title chosen by the artist, and on many there is a supplementary note which he has engraved or written into the margin. In this series there are groups with sexual content, as, for example, *Bien tirada ésta* (Stylish Dressing), in which the girl is dressing up with the assistance of a bawd. In the *¡Que Sacrificio!* (What a Sacrifice!) old roués in lascivious attitudes and with lecherous glances surround a young girl. Another group has themes which are social or political; donkeys ride on poor Spaniards, for example, or a monkey and an ass are doctor and patient. Finally, Goya included some very strange designs of demons and witches collecting in wild flight, killing their sacrifices, plucking out their feathers and even their genitals. The title-engraving is also phantastic: Goya is surrounded by spirits, one of whom is handing him a pen so that he can draw them. The title he has written is "The sleep of reason produced monsters."

He emerged from his seclusion and later, in 1798, he painted the frescoes for the chapel of Sta Antonia de la Florida, finishing them in three months. In composition they once more resemble the earlier and attractive genre-pictures, but the choice of theme, and the half-decayed corpse (St. Anthony reviving a dead man), are reminiscent of the unpleasant experiences depicted in the "Caprichos". Apparently Goya could not escape from these experiences, or so, at least, it is suggested by his pictures of the year 1798; for example, "Carnival", "The Procession of Flagellants", "The Tribunal of the Inquisition", "The Madhouse".

At this time he was becoming deaf, an affliction which grew still worse later on. About this time, also, his one great love, the Infanta Alba, died suddenly. Europe was now in trouble, and in Spain, church, civic rights and morality all showed signs of decay. In France, Napoleon's star was rising, and in 1808 the French seized the government of Spain; the horrors of war began. Goya retreated to his newly-built country house, living in the greatest isolation. Here he worked at a fresh series of etchings, "Los desastres de la guerra" ("The Disasters of the War"), and adorned the walls of his room with frescoes, from which ghosts, demons, witches, vampires and murder all stared down at him. The new etchings are symbolic compositions with strange animal shapes, and realistic scenes of war. In the "With or without Reason", for instance, an overwhelming French force is shooting down a few poor Spanish peasants. In another the subject is reversed; its title is "There is No Difference". In several designs there are mangled corpses, or violated dead women lie under the ruins of houses. Finally, in one design, a man vomits over a heap of dead: *¿Para eso habeis nacido?* (Were Ye Born For This?). "Los desastres de la guerra" were succeeded by the series "Los Proverbios", designed in 1814–1815. Other authors call the "Proverbios": "Sueños" or "Dreams". Apart from one which is inscribed "Disparate Claro" ("Clear Confusion"), these are not named, and for the most part the "Proverbios" have been given inadequate titles by art critics whose interpretations conflict. Some of the designs show more comprehensible motifs, as, for example, the puppet-show; others are full of ghost-shapes, beings with divided bodies, legs, mixtures of men and women. The "Proverbios" impress one as dark, dismal, repellent and incomprehensible.

About 1817 Goya left his isolation to travel to Seville; at that time he completed his "Tauromachia" or bullfighting designs. Once more he worked on religious pictures, portraits and the like, which betray a quiet seriousness and a sincere belief; the colours are subdued. His new genre pictures, such as the "Women at the Fountain", once again show beautiful form and colouring. In 1824 the old man, now aged seventy-eight, was again in flight; this time the reason is supposedly the anger aroused by a drawing with political reference. However, nothing certain is known, and Goya soon returned to Spain. Then, in spite of being highly honoured both by the public and the king, he went back once more to France, where he died in 1828 of apoplexy.

Several elements in Goya's life-history may point to pathological trends. First, his frequent flights, which continued till his old age. For these restless escapades the documentary evidence is insufficient and contradictory. His first flight has been explained as due to the attentions of the Inquisition, the second as due to the attentions of the police. Yet these reasons are frequently confused chronologically. The flight from Italy was romantically explained, but vaguely like the reasons ("on political grounds") given for his flight in 1824. We may note that he returned direct from Rome to Zaragoza from which he had had to flee, six years earlier, so we are told, from the Inquisition. And one may legitimately wonder why a man under the ban of the Inquisition and of the police should be protected by the Spanish ambassador and allowed to travel without fear of consequences from Italy back to Spain. Goya soon returned from his political flight—an indication of how much credence one may give to the cause.

Secondly, Goya's fairly sudden "retirements". We know little about them, but their motivation appears to be psycho-pathological. Though his first withdrawal was attributed by some biographers to his idyllic seclusion with the Infanta Alba, Goya about this time wrote to one of his friends saying: "My health is just as it was. I am frequently so excited that I cannot endure myself." Three months after this letter he wrote to Bernardo Yriarte, on January 4, 1794, ". . . to occupy the imaginative power deadened by so much brooding over my pain". Such evidence suggests that his condition was one in which periods of excitement alternated with morbid brooding. His second "retirement" only appears to have been caused by outside events; in fact, it had nothing to do with politics, since both the Spanish and the French esteemed him. He was so submissive to the French that, as Calvert relates, he helped Napoli and Maella to select the fifty best pictures from the royal gallery for dispatch to the Louvre. It is hard to reconcile this with feelings of patriotism. Moreover, his seclusion had nothing to do with the war, the horrors of which began in 1808, whereas it was not until 1811–12 that he withdrew into retirement. No documents exist about this period of his life, and consequently, his seclusion remains mysterious for his biographers.

A third pathological element in Goya's life-history is this: that, even if one allows for the fact that Goya was an artist of the Late Spanish Rococo and held standards of conduct appropriate to the period, he behaved pathologically. His adventures appear to have been unscrupulous, and his love, which he experienced only at a mature period of his life, he took as a great opportunity for boasting. He was querulous and belligerent. In a letter from Zaragoza, dated March 18, 1781, he wrote at great length to the Building Committee. Scornfully and insolently he criticized the objections to his sketches, boasted repeatedly that he was a member of the Royal Academy, that the royal family was enchanted by him and that all his pictures had been received with great acclamation. He complained that intrigues were being conducted against him, that his enemies were dragging his private life into a blaze of publicity just to set the public against him. He considered that the committee were biased, for they mentioned only the faults in his work. Bayeau had already seen his plans; why was it only now that he objected to the pictures? Goya would not care to assert that it was being done intentionally in order to ruin him as an artist, for he had not sufficient proof—etc. Undoubtedly he did have difficulties with the Building Committee, but if one compares the way in which other artists, for example, those of the Renaissance, reacted in similar circumstances, one will see that Goya's reactions on what was, after all, a comparatively trivial occasion, were almost paranoid.

To sum up these indications, Goya's life-history shows flights of obscure motivation, when he is restless, bumptious and over-active; in contrast it shows at least two retirements of equally obscure motivation, when he is deadened, withdrawn and full of pain. These swings of mood can plausibly be evaluated as expression of an illness of the manic-depressive type. If one makes use of the crude body-type theory of Kretschmer, Goya's constitution—so far as can be judged from portraits, including the one by himself—was of the pyknic variety, which would also favour the diagnosis of a manic-depressive psychosis. His death from apoplexy, a disease characteristic both of pyknics and of manic-depressives, points in the same direction. In accordance with this, in his elated mood his pictures are of pleasant colouring and are descriptive and realistic, features stated by Kretschmer to be typical of the cyclothymes.

Yet several aspects contradict this diagnosis. Goya's personality before his illness was querulous and belligerent; his family life was unhappy and badly organized; he died in a foreign country. A cyclothyme would have arranged all that far better and would have been able to find more harmony in life. His unpatriotic act in helping Napoli and Maella to send away the best pictures to France suggests emotional detachment rather than depression. Furthermore, Goya's prolific output is against the diagnosis of depression. In all, Goya produced about seventeen hundred works of art, of which about six hundred belong to the period of his illness. One-third of all his production, therefore, was created during his illness; such a creative productivity is never seen in melancholia. One could, moreover, consider his flights as expressions of a psycho-pathological "wanderlust" or, in other words, as expressions of a schizophrenic dromomania and his retirements as autistic periods; this would indicate the diagnosis of a schizophrenic reaction. Goya's pre-morbid personality and especially his paranoid trends are well in accordance with this tentative diagnosis.

More decisive support is given to a diagnosis of schizophrenia by the designs he made during his autistic periods. A very brief indication of their appearance has already been offered. So far as content is concerned it appears that they are "romantic" or phantastic rather than descriptive and realistic. But closer examination of these etchings reveals some features of greater diagnostic importance. The "Caprichos" and the "Sueños" have only vague contact with external reality; they depict the inner experiences of Goya, and the engraving "Sopla" (Fig. 14) indicates the kind of experiences they were. At this period the belief in witches had disappeared from Spain and witch-hunts no longer took place; consequently the source of the theme is endogenous to the artist. "Ya tienen asiento" is almost vulgar and very crude in its sexuality; the symbolic factors in it are dominant, just as they are in the picture of the metamorphosed doctor and patient and in all the others as well. The "Proverbios" show a still more marked alienation from reality, representing a world of pure phantasy. They depict disturbed spatial relations and they show obvious displacement and pictorial condensation; in them body-parts are cut off, multiplied and divided. In Fig. 15, for instance, detached heads with chattering teeth give melody to the rhythm of the castanets; the discrepancy in the size and grouping of the figures suggests unreality. In Plate 16, instead of detached body parts, multiplication of body parts is depicted: heads are doubled, the man in the foreground seems to have four arms, and there are displacements of body-parts. Reality and unreality lose their boundaries. Fig. 16 shows in abundance pictorial condensation of the shapes of men and women or human and animal into one. Compositions of such a kind, which I have already discussed in Chapter 3, are *pathognomonic* of schizophrenic experiences.

Goya's illness also finds expression in the titles of his engravings and in his subsequent attitude towards them. Each picture of the "Caprichos" has a title, which is organically linked to the design in a way similar to that "writing in" of schizophrenic drawings discussed in Chapter 2. The inscription on the title page as originally planned by Goya has been noted. Another etching Goya merely called "Tooth Hunting"; this depicts a disgusting

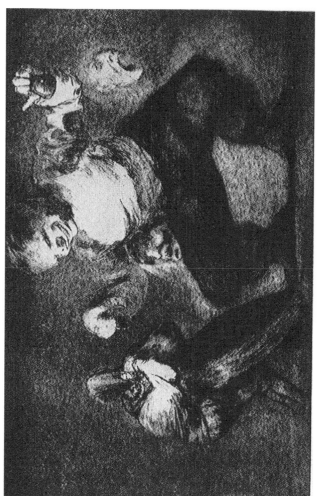

Fig. 15. Goya: Plate 26 of the Caprichos

face p. 150

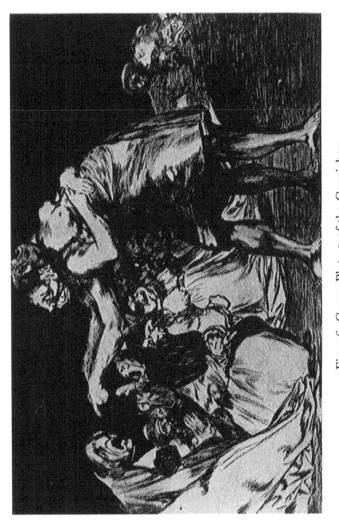

Fig. 16. Goya: Plate 7 of the Caprichos

and fearful scene. When recovering from his illness, however, Goya dallied over the publication of his "Caprichos"; and before they were published he made alterations in the titles. On the title leaf he wrote "Phantasy without reason produces monstrosities; purified, however, they bring forth true art and create wonder". Ultimately he replaced the title page with a rather unimaginative self-portrait. Under the "Tooth Hunting" he wrote: "Is it not pitiful that people still believe in such stupidities?" The superficiality of those remarks in no way harmonizes with the pictures and the original titles; it is possible to explain this by the fact that after his illness Goya no longer could understand them completely. They were alien to him because their function was anchored in his illness, which, when he had recovered from it, became to him incomprehensible; hence he tried to rationalize the documents of his illness with titles, which would restore contact with reality once more. Goya's retrospective attitude to his engravings, this subsequent lack of understanding, so it seems, of his own work, corresponds more to what we see in schizophrenics than in manic-depressives. Present-day developments in psychiatry have blurred many of the former diagnostic entities; often it would be hair-splitting to discuss whether a case should be labelled recurrent schizophrenia or manic-depressive psychosis with schizophrenic features. What seems to be significant is that those aspects of Goya's work which are aesthetically incomprehensible can be readily understood when psychiatric considerations are introduced. At that point the interpretative and speculative work of the pathographer is concluded. However, it would be alluring to extend the ideas developed in the previous chapter to this examination of Goya. Some of the designs, such as Plate 5, of the "Proverbios", deliberately convey loss of boundaries between reality and unreality and alterations in the temporal system; others depict marked disturbances of the body image and the spatial system. But because we lack an adequate clinical history such a commentary must reluctantly be abandoned.

11

III

The power of illness to modify art by causing alterations in style and content is only one of the problems
arising from such studies as I have outlined above. The
psycho-pathological schools have been interested in ascer-
taining how far art products, modified through illness,
have a function for the artist himself. But so far, those
studies have led to conclusions applicable to anyone at
all who ever did some painting before his illness, that is
to say, to anyone who displayed some degree of craftsmanship. Quite another problem is posed when the individual
who maintained productivity throughout his illness was a
creative artist such as Goya.

To draw satisfactory inference from a pathography one
must consider personality, art and illness as a whole. In
consequence the question arises, To what extent does an
illness in a creative artist become transformed, modified
or merely reduced in its severity by means of his art?
This is an interesting problem in research which calls for
special investigations outside the scope of my present
inquiry. Further problems, aesthetic and sociological,
arise out of the pathographies: how far have the art products of morbid artists furthered the development of art
and influenced cultural advancement? Maudsley formulated his answer in a positive sense when he said, "What
right have we to believe Nature under any sort of obliga-
tion to do her work by means of complete minds only?
She may find an incomplete mind a more suitable
instrument for a particular purpose."

VIII

CULTURAL INFLUENCES

Art as an expression of culture and its influence upon it—Art as a means of psycho-therapy.

I

THE APPEARANCES, MECHANISMS, dynamics and motivations of schizophrenic paintings have been analysed, all, so far, in relation to the endogenous, that is internal, biological factors. Exogenous, that is to say, environmental or cultural, influences should play an equally important part in the analysis. Unfortunately, at present, we lack comparative material. The paintings of Western European schizophrenics do not show marked differences as far as cultural influences are concerned, and schizophrenic paintings from America as reproduced by A. Rosanoff do not appear to be different from the European paintings reproduced by Prinzhorn. If they were available, schizophrenic paintings executed by patients of a more markedly different cultural background, e.g. Indian or Chinese, would offer the basis for a comparative analysis.

But there is another problem in this matter of environmental influences. It has been mentioned that there exist numerous similarities between schizophrenic and "modern" art products, though these similarities are only apparent. The dynamics of modern painting can be shown to be those of a conscious and deliberate analysis. The question then arises: what are the cultural factors which move the modern artist to produce paintings with resemblance at least to the work of the schizophrenic patient?

To apply to these cultural factors a psycho-physiological viewpoint does not help very much. Brickner, for instance, emphasizes the cognitive aspect of culture. He calls attention to the concept of telencephalization, that is, the functional dominance of the roof brain over the rest of the nervous system, and goes on to state that culture is its expression. In his words, "acculturation (in giving form to telencephalization) operates in the service of survival functions because the function of telencephalization is to produce increasingly elaborate means for their expression". As the cortex matures, the material for learning becomes more abundant; this is essential for the process of telencephalization. The material comes mainly from cultural sources and is learned from the parents. Masserman, on the other hand, does not restrict his interest to the way in which culture expresses telencephalization, but links the two systems more dynamically. He emphasizes, in an over-simplified way, that all human activity is directed towards the satisfaction of physiological *needs*. He specifies the physiological viewpoint in his "principle of substitutive adaptation", which states: "When the direct satisfaction of some combination of physiological needs becomes difficult or impossible, behaviour becomes deviated into indirect channels of goal-seeking, or is diverted towards the satisfaction of other combinations of need." In such a system, art plays a dual role: (*a*) it influences the various patterns of behaviour, that is, signs acquire "meaning"; and (*b*) these meanings can be drastically altered by subsequent experiences. These biological aspects re-emphasize the cognitive and biological nature of culture generally and of art particularly. They also demonstrate the significance of cognitive factors in moulding our environment, and emphasize the weakness of too sharp a dichotomy between the intrinsic and the extrinsic determinants of behaviour.

Thus in the analysis of cultural influences we have to consider other ways of approach. The anthropological method has often been used, but its scope is limited just as the psychophysiological method is limited. Anthropological formulations refer only to the patterns of primitive culture: they cannot be applied without considerable modification to complex communities such as our own. The misunderstandings that arise from applying anthropological concepts in too simple a form lead to such a conclusion for example as that "our whole way of life and thought is breaking down", or, as the poet Robert Graves has expanded it, that poets and artists become to some extent dissociated from the social order in which they live, and "exiled in the wilderness". Thus in their work they do not express any cultural values but experiment in various ways with form devoid of content. Graves has stated in *The White Goddess*: "It is not as though the so-called surrealists, impressionists, expressionists and neo-romantics were concealing a grand secret by pretended folly . . . on the contrary, they are concealing their unhappy lack of a secret." The critic Raymond Mortimer also believes in a gulf between the public and the painter, owing to the painter's voluntary exile; he thinks that to-day's art contains no communication, and for the lack of it, it has lost its *raison d'être*. According to Mortimer, a religious revival might stem this rapid decline in pictorial art. Some of the modern artists themselves feel isolated. Paul Klee exclaimed, "We still lack the ultimate power, for the people are not with us."

So it appears necessary to apply sociological definitions and in this manner to differentiate between "civilization" which involves utilitarianism, and "culture" which is the sum total of non-utilitarian activities. The interaction of both has been subject to various investigations, but here only a broad and necessarily brief outline will be given in support of my main theme. It will be best to compare two racially and geographically distinct cultures and their artistic expression; for this reason the Chinese and the Western European have been chosen.

Chinese painting in its origin was part of a religious ritual and as such entirely of secondary value, but later it became, through the needs and wishes of the court, of primary value. Its subsequent history shows how various military conquests, religious and political changes, altered the pattern of Chinese painting. Up to this point, both Eastern and Western art had shown a parallelism in their development, but a few peculiarities of Chinese painting may be noted. It was more or less a secret craft handed down from father to son. Essentially it was a strongly formal and traditional mode of expression; once a motif had been established it was faithfully copied for centuries. These motifs were of representational nature, but tended strongly to develop a symbolic content as well. The picture of a bird, for instance, a flower, or an animal, in Chinese painting was used also to suggest another meaning; thus the picture of a bat suggested also happiness and "plum flower" also represented female beauty. Hence, pictorial combinations such as geese and bamboo acquired well-established symbolic meanings which were always employed in the same context. But, as S. Yenyns has shown, whereas the social environment underwent alterations the pictorial motifs owing to the marked traditionalism in painting remained the same, and ultimately became signs without content. This was so much the case that the meaning of most of the motifs became incomprehensible to scholars themselves. The symbols apparently became conventionalized.

Nevertheless, if geese and bamboo stand for proverbial religious and philosophical values, they cannot be a special bamboo or the representation of some particular goose, but they have to reproduce *the* bamboo and *the* goose to fulfil their general symbolic role. E. Newton expressed this by saying that the Chinese artist paints the essence and not the existence; he paints what he *knows* and not what he actually sees. When the Chinese paints a landscape his attempt is not to give his personal perception of the landscape, but the generalized conception, the idea of that landscape. Whether traditionalism is an expression of this search for the universal, or whether the detached search for truth is a factor moulding Chinese culture in general, is less relevant than the fact that the interaction has produced the peculiar pictorial art of the Chinese.

The Western artist on the other hand, once he became a creator of primary values, painted what he saw and not what is known. Both in Western and in Eastern painting, needless to say, the emergence of art as a primary value entailed the development of pattern and formal restructuring for their own sake. In both there was an interplay between tendencies to exact representation and tendencies to patterning, with the emphasis now going in one direction and now in the other. In both the ways in which artists formulate their aims and intentions cannot always be accepted at their face value, but often require interpretation or restatement in accordance with modern psychological and aesthetic knowledge. The manner in which pictorial art emerged as a primary value in the two cultures, the detailed differences in the development of structural principles, the dynamic interaction of tendencies in the contrasted cultures are matters for the art historian which I cannot pursue here. It will be sufficient to note that in Western painting the artist concerned himself with the re-structuring of a particular presented situation; in Asiatic art as a rule he concerns himself with the structuring of a generalized or conceptual situation. The Western painter, then, interested himself in the actual appearance of a particular thing, attempting to give his own re-structured perception of it. His main interest was the appearance of his surroundings and not the essence of them. But this attitude does not imply, as E. Newton assumes, that once artists achieved their freedom from control by social forces such as the church, the state, etc., they became individualistic to an extreme degree. The products of the Western artist have always expressed the cultural values of his time. For instance, photography has taught us that when the galloping horse has its fore legs extended, its hind legs are brought underneath

the body. Through this *knowledge* our perceptual appreciation of Georgian sporting prints with their long-drawn
horses has altered; the galloping horses in them do not
nowadays suggest speed to artists or to onlookers. A new
way of pictorial representation began through this knowledge, as R. Wilenski demonstrated.

An indirect interrelation between civilization and art
is the civilized creation of the machine. It is logical, as
H. Read has pointed out, that the art of the machine-age
should not be naturalistic, but is bound to become
"abstract", an art of geometrical proportions and purely
formal harmonies. Again, the twentieth century has seen
the popular rise of psycho-analytic doctrine. Its elaboration into our cultural theme became manifest in the
surrealist movement, which chose as its sole subject-
matter—the subconscious. The intellectual interest stimu-
lated by Freud's teachings turned towards the art products
of psychotic artists; Goya was looked upon by art historians as one who did not fit into the spirit of his period,
Blake as an isolated phenomenon, and Grünewald for
unknown reasons as a simultaneous mixture of the past
Gothic and of the coming Baroque; the work of these
artists became appreciated and understood through the
stimulation of a new interest and they began to influence
modern painters. Such examples, chosen at random, all
reflect, as H. Read has emphasized, the various cultural
trends within our society. From another point of view
Waddington has drawn attention to the rapidity of
modern life, which does not allow enough time to assimi-
late problems and get an accepted artistic solution for
them. But in spite of the complexity of the appearances,
of the subject-matter chosen, the main Western cultural
tendency, that is, a subjective interest in life, has remained
the same. This common factor in Western art seems the
more important when it is contrasted with Eastern art
as outlined here. Furthermore, it appears that "modern"
artists display an analytical interest in life, becoming
more objective than subjective, or, as E. Newton calls it,
they become puritanistic. Thus the seeming similarities

between schizophrenic and "modern" art in no way indicate a dissolution of our culture, but reflect a phase of dynamic cultural development.

Above, by treating culture in sociological terms, I have indicated that an artist, even in our complex culture, is never divorced from his background. McIver, on the other hand, differentiates culture from civilization by arguing that whilst the character of civilization is standardization, that of culture is individualism, and the active function of the latter lies in operating by its individualistic impact on the former. A similar viewpoint has been emphasized by Lord Russell in his Reith Lectures.

Of the active functions of art in the community, a few should be enumerated here. First, pictorial art can on occasions be more effective than language, a fact which has been analysed by Masserman. Pictorial representations in political or commercial propaganda or the cartoons of our time would illustrate this. Secondly, art is said to have the capacity of graduating emotions. In this respect art functions in a utilitarian manner in relation to society. The graduation of emotion is achieved through the aesthetic experience, which according to Bullough is based on the factor of physical distance. Without this, art would be too personal and the emotional release too explosive. Thus, watching a drama, we identify ourselves with the hero and work out our conflicts through this identification, not being aware that it is our conflict we are releasing. Identification is probably self-evident in such an example as that which I have just given, but this identification (empathy) is a less satisfactory postulate when pictorial art has to be considered. For in what sense can empathy explain the aesthetic enjoyment of a male spectator looking at Giorgone's "Venus", if aphrodisiacal components are evidently excluded? If the man identifies himself with the figure, this makes sense only to a psycho-analytic evaluator (hidden homosexuality) or to an "analytical psychologist" (anima projection). Clearly empathy fails on many other occasions to explain aesthetic responses. Nevertheless, Bullough's theory is still accepted by many investigators as a working hypothesis in the study of the social aspects of art.

Aesthetic experience demands as a *sine qua non* that one has to "understand the picture one looks at". One appreciates a picture; whether appreciation has an emotional component or not, it can only be possible if the formal pattern present in the picture is comprehended by the onlooker. In a historical perspective one can safely state that as far as art expresses dominant and prevalent cultural factors, aesthetic appreciation is unhampered. The incongruity arises when the artist, through his individuality, differs from the social background and employs new and hitherto not accepted methods. With many of the pictorial art products of present-day creative artists the technique involved is such that the painting cannot be understood by a large number of the onlookers. The artists have attempted to visualize in a direction which is not that of the established contemporary vision. Nevertheless, they have re-moulded our appreciation of patterns in art. Contemporary art demands—according to its nature—a more marked intellectual collaboration in appreciating it. This intellectualization of aesthetic experiences has allowed a perceptual appreciation of patterns suggestive of schizophrenia, especially when the painting is in the form of posters, advertisements, etc.— Waddington expresses this wittily: "The man in the Tube may never have seen a picture by Picasso, and if he did might dislike it; but he would not regard it with quite the same blank incomprehension or shocked hatred as did his father, who had never sat opposite a watered-down Picasso advising him to "Go By Underground—It's Quicker." In such a sense, art exerts yet another active function.

II

When one is reviewing the social functions of art its therapeutic and educative properties have to be considered as well. The utilization of art for educative purposes has been attempted and advocated from various aspects. It is evident that as this study concerns itself with psychotic art, a review of therapeutic attempts is more justified than one of educative or "preventative" efforts. On the other hand, some mention of the latter is indicated, when the social implications are discussed.

Educative problems are intimately connected with children's art. To treat the subject-matter appropriately one should correlate the psycho-physiological development of children with the nature of their particular cultural background; one should relate development in drawing to the special characteristics of the growing mind; one should outline the special world of the child; one should especially investigate children with ability in craftsmanship, and one should take into account the pre-existing trends of teaching in craftsmanship and so forth. It is apparent that such a treatment demands a study of its own. Herbert Read in his *Education through Art* has attempted a synthesis of the various aspects of "children's art" that I have enumerated. He has drawn attention to the importance of sensation and built up a theory which attempts to show that if in the upbringing of children the vividness of their sensations is preserved by certain recommended methods, as a result more satisfactory human interrelations may develop. "Idealism would then no longer be an escape from reality; it would be a simple human response to reality." As *Education through Art* is one of the most significant works of the past few years, it has to be more closely examined. The synthesis and the methods of education recommended by Read are based on anatomical, physiological and psychological evidence, much of which shows serious shortcomings. A few of these should be enumerated here. Read accepts that "the analysis of the structure of the brain suggests the possibility of a physical location for the three levels into which Freud divided the mental personality, the id, the ego and the super-ego". Now, as I mentioned in the introduction, mental manifestations have no direct relation to structure, but to the function of that structure. Furthermore, the terms, super-ego, ego and id denote hypothetical concepts which may offer a working hypothesis for a dynamic psychology; but to search for their cerebral location is incorrect.

Psychologically, *Education through Art* accepts the ideas of the Gestalt school including that of isomorphism, which correlates phenomenal experience with structural events. This, from a psychophysiological viewpoint, may be correct, but the anatomical and physiological basis of it is outdated. Anatomically Kohler argued that configurations are perceived as such in the calcarine part of the cerebral cortex, whereas the evidence indicates that there is a separate demonstrable centre with visuo-gnostic function, that is, it enables what is seen to be understood. In other words, this centre has synthetic or configurational functions, elaborating the amorphous material that is registered by the calcarine cortex. The "electrostatic patterns" of the isomorphists cannot be confirmed by electro-encephalographic studies. Furthermore, the formulation that "chemical reactions accompany nervous activity" is incorrect; nervous activity can be *expressed* in biochemical terms, as Sir Henry Dale and his collaborators have shown, or it can be expressed in electrophysiological terms. These two modes of approach are complementary to one another, and both are modes of evaluation of nervous activity. On the purely psychological side B. Peterman's work still represents the basic critical survey of Kohler's ideas. Thus the theoretical background of Read's synthesis needs re-examination, but his statement of problems should stimulate further investigations into his very important inquiry—how far, that is, can art as an educative means alter human behaviour?

As I have said, the therapeutic possibilities of art closely concern this study of schizophrenic art. Art as a psychotherapeutic means has a long history; it has been employed from various viewpoints with various techniques. Although every division is somewhat artificial, leaving out one aspect or the other and simplifying unjustifiably, I would be inclined for the sake of brevity to review in such a simplified manner the various approaches to the therapeutic use of art. A detailed review would call for a monograph of its own.

Art as a hobby was recommended by psycho-therapists before the establishment of the current psychopathological schools. Its subjects were mostly the neurotic type of patients, only some of whom bordered on psychosis. Its technique was the teaching of craftsmanship largely along naturalistic lines. Sometimes it achieved its aim in helping the patient to develop a certain degree of technique. But it was seldom used for purposes of proper self-expression, and it furthered an undesirable dilettantism. In fact, it was a kind of occupational therapy: it had nothing to do with art.

Art as a psycho-therapeutic auxiliary was introduced by the pupils of Freud. Pictorial symbols were looked upon in the same way as dream products, namely, as the disguised expression of thoughts which had to be interpreted and ultimately verbalized. It was to be expected, verbalization being the ultimate aim, that the paintings collected by Freudians would exclusively be children's paintings—Jung's mystical approach was more successful in furthering the pictorial expression of adults. Yet the pictures so obtained have no originality, since both their appearance and content are of a suggested nature (see p. 136).

The encouragement of spontaneous self-expression is yet another organized method of art treatment, much under discussion in England at the present time. Lectures on art followed by the encouragement of spontaneous drawings were originated during the war by the British Red Cross, and the method found its way to the psychiatric institutions. Fundamentally, the method is twofold; first the lectures on pictorial art and then the formation of art classes in which, under the direction of an art teacher, the patients paint whatever they wish. The art teacher is merely an expert who encourages, but does not *teach* technique. Two types of such art classes seem to emerge, largely depending on the art masters. In the one type, the art master is unable to suppress his own personality and thus influences his class. This alters the class in that the talented patients become active and their pictorial products improve in quality, though to a great degree they reflect the art master's personality and approach to art. The other type of art class develops a less homogeneous character in its product, owing to the fact that the master successfully maintains a negative personality in the particular situation. The utility of art classes is partly diagnostic, partly therapeutic by the encouragement of self-expression; they will be therapeutically useful only if the art master refrains from teaching craftsmanship.

But they enjoy one more characteristic in contrast to the more individual methods I have mentioned: the classes give rise to more material than can be obtained through individual encouragement. This provokes an important question, namely, whether or no there are some group dynamics present in those art classes, which influence the superior quality and greater quantity of the art products? I have raised this question in previous publications and since made some observations on painting classes where male and female patients, hospitalized neurotics and psychotics, worked together. The studio, paints, brushes, stands, etc., were a change after the rest of the hospital environment. The patients arrived individually, and took generally a stereotyped choice of place, e.g. the same corner in the studio; they talked now and then to their neighbour or neighbours, but no further intimacy with the rest of the class developed. They did not show an interest in the drawings of others, nor in the fate of their work when accomplished, that is, of their completed painting.

This short description would suggest that group dynamics are only minimally present in the art classes of psychiatric institutions. In a group, members enter into distinct relations, into functional interconnections; they develop common attitudes; they develop traditions and so forth. None of these are present in the art classes; they are merely classes or, in the sociological term, associations. Associations consist of interest-conscious units, with no definite organization, the emphasis being on the "interest" in contradistinction to the "attitude" of a group. As McIver puts it, "We cultivate an art . . . and find it desirable to join with others in so doing." Thus there is a tendency to form associations and the satisfaction of this tendency may be the explanation of the greater productivity of those art classes, reinforcing the drive for spontaneous individual self-expression in painting. On the other hand, such art classes do not give an impetus to modifying human interrelations within a diagnostically inhomogeneous crowd of patients.

American experiments, however, have gone further, though detailed reports are still not available. One group therapist let his group become "integrated". Once his crowd became a group, he gave them the task of painting a mural together. Out of such a task two possibilities may arise; first, a diagnostic one, namely, how far an integrated group is able to organize a picture; or, in other words, the mural becomes an objective measure of the group integration. Secondly, it might well be that the common task of painting a mural gives a further impetus to group integration. If this can be shown affirmatively, then the sociological query of whether "art is an integrative force" might be answered as well. Naturally, the first control experiment required is to prove whether any other task would integrate a group equally well; if it would not, then it would seem more probable that art has a positive integrative force within a group. The question of the socially integrative force of art is the point where this discussion of art as a therapeutic means links up with the rest of the problem of the present chapter.

Before concluding, however, something needs to be said about the value of all these art therapies. The diagnostic value of spontaneous products is immense, and any means (art classes, etc.) which encourages this is welcome. So many latent schizophrenias, well controlled by the personality, become unveiled through painting. Thus it is, in a sense, a "projective technique" of the diagnostic armory. It also offers possibilities for various experimental investigations such as the investigation reported by E. C. Dax at the meeting of the British Council of Rehabilitation; Dax allowed his patients to paint under controlled conditions whilst playing classical music to them. The paintings show some uniformity, conditioned by the stimulus rather than by the mental state of the patients. It is too early, however, to comment on his findings. T. Greene has reviewed similar investigations, and H. Sigerist has commented on these problems from a therapeutic point of view as well.

As an occupational therapy at a higher level, art treatment is to be encouraged, but as a treatment *per se* it does not seem to have much value. Whether a patient acts out his "autistic phantasies" in artistic creation and gets better by means of this, is highly questionable; the duty of the psychiatrist is in the first instance to help and not to rely on chance therapeutic results. Hence he will reinforce his physical methods of treatment with encouragement to paint, and *vice versa*. No psychotic on record has been cured by means of painting alone; this, of course, excludes the true artists whose relationship to their art, including the question of the healing value of their art, has already been raised. But this specific question at present has to remain unanswered.

SUMMARY

THE JUSTIFICATION OF a survey of psychotic art lies in the employment of a different viewpoint. This in the present survey is the psycho-physiological viewpoint, from which all mental manifestations are seen as related to cerebral function; cerebral function in its turn is related to structure. Such a viewpoint assesses art as a manifestation of man's cognitive capability.

Psychotic art, especially schizophrenic art, has been studied as far as its appearance is concerned, and it has been shown that several of the schizophrenic patternings are physiologically conditioned. Supporting evidence has been sought not only through clinical observations but also from experimental results, such as the mescalin investigations.

The content of schizophrenic paintings is determined by the peculiarities in the mental life of the schizophrenics. Of these peculiarities, the body image disturbances seem of crucial importance, as they reflect on disturbed categorical (time and space) experiences. Furthermore, the body image is a better operational term than the hypothetical "ego". It has been shown how far schizophrenic art is influenced through disturbances of the body image on the basis of experimental and clinical evidence.

The disturbed categorical thinking of the schizophrenic artists suggested the examination of the cognitive aspect of art, which has been to a certain degree investigated by several workers. It has been found that factors which acutely alter the categorical thinking, such as an injury to the brain, induce alterations in pictorial appearances

12

similar to those of schizophrenics. The nature of these cognitive alterations has been more closely scrutinized and it has been suggested that the so-called categorical or abstract and situational or concrete attitudes are not necessarily antagonistic, but that in artists they may be simultaneously present. A hypothesis of such a simultaneous presence of the two "basic modes of psychological existence" in artists has been expanded.

Of the dynamics of psychotic art, the explanations of the various psychopathological schools (Freud and Jung) and of typologists have been scrutinized.

Yet another aspect of the dynamics lies in environmental factors. Cultural influences on schizophrenic paintings are unexplored; an attempt has been made, however, to examine cultural factors which influence "modern" artists to paint schizophrenic-like pictures. It has been emphasized that the similarities of schizophrenic and modern art are only apparent because the attitude of modern painters is deliberately analytical, which always results in some seeming fragmentation, and because modern art is a logical consequence of cultural events.

Psychotic art involves the question of art-therapy; a review of this, however, offers little which would justify an organization of it in a broader sense.

Throughout this study it has been emphasized that whilst the aspect employed is a specific one, the points raised and the conclusions drawn do not claim to offer a generalized theory. The cognitive components are merely *components* of psychotic or non-psychotic art. But it is better to arrive at some truth even if it represents only a fraction of the vast problem of art. "The problem"—to use Sherrington's words—"has one virtue at least, it will long offer to those who pursue it the comfort that to journey is better than to arrive . . . and when that arrival comes, there may be regret that the pursuit is over."

BIBLIOGRAPHY

Adrian, E. D. *The Basis of Sensation*. Norton, New York, 1928.

Adrian, E. D. "Electrical Activities of the Nervous System." *Arch. Neurol. Psych.*, vol. 38, p. 1125, 1934.

Anastasi, A., and Foley, T. "Survey of the Literature on Artistic Behaviour of the Abnormal." *J. Gen. Psychol.*, vol. 25, p. 187, 1940.

Anastasi, A., and Foley, T. "A Survey of the Literature on Artistic Behaviour in the Abnormal." *Psychological Monographs*, vol. 52, 1940.

Bartlett, F. C. *Psychology and Primitive Culture*. Cambridge, 1923.

Baynes, H. G. *Mythology of the Soul*. London, 1923.

Bender, L. "Psychoses Associated with Somatic Diseases that Distort Body Structure." *Arch. Neurol. and Psych.*, vol. 32, p. 1000, 1934.

Bender, L. "Visual Motor Gestalt Test and its Clinical Use." *Res. Monogr. Amer. Orthopsych.* New York, 1938.

Benedict, R. *Patterns of Culture*. Routledge, London, 1946.

Boas, F. *General Anthropology*. Heath, Boston, 1938.

Brain, W. R. "Visual Disorientation with Special Reference to Lesions of the Right Cerebral Hemisphere." *Brain*, vol. 44, p. 244, 1941.

Brickner, R. M. *Telencephalization (in Frontal Lobes)*. Williams and Wilkins, Baltimore, 1948.

Burt, Sir Cyril. *Mental and Scholastic Tests*. Staples Press, Ltd., London, 2nd ed., 1947.

Bychowsky, G. "The Body Image." *Journ. Nerv. & Mental Disease*, vol. 97, 1943.

Cameron, N. "Reasoning, Regression and Communication in Schizophrenics." *Psychol. Monograph.*, No. 50, 1938.

Cameron, N. "The Functional Psychosis," Chapter 29, or *Personality and Behaviour Disorders*. Ronald Press, New York, 1944.

Chweitzer, A., Geblewicz, E., and Liberson, W. "Action of Mescaline on the Alpha Waves." *Compt. Rend. Soc. Biol.*, vol. 124, p. 1206, 1937.

Cox, J. W. *Mechanical Aptitude, its Existence, Nature and Measurement*. Methuen, London, 1928.

Dalbiez, E. *Psychoanalytical Methods and the Doctrine of Freud*. Longmans, London, 1941.

Dali, Salvador. *La Conquête de l'irrationel*. Editions Surréalistes, Paris, 1935.

Durkheim, E. *The Rules of Sociologic Method*. Chicago University Press, 1938.

Earle, F. M., and Gaw, F. *The Measurement of Manual Dexterities*. Nat. Inst. of Ind. Psycho., London, 1930.

Evans, J. *Taste and Temperament*. Cape, London, 1939.

Eysenck, H. J. *Dimensions of Personality*. Kegan Paul, London, 1947.

Eysenck, H. J. "Experimental Study of the Good Gestalt." *Psychol. Rev.*, No. 49, 1942.

Forster, E. "Selbstversuch mit Meskalin." *Zschr. ges. Neurol. & Psych.*, vol. 46, 1919.

Freeman, F. N. "An Experimental Study of Handwriting." *Psych. Mongr.*, 1914.

Freeman, F. N. *Psychology of the Common Branches*. Harrap, London, 1916.

Freud, S. *Collected Papers*. Inter. Psychoanal. Library, Hogarth, London, 1945.

Goldstein, K., and Gelb, A. "Psychologische Analysen hirnpathologische Falle." *Zschr. f.d. ges. Neurol. v. Psychiat.*, 41 Pl., 1918.

Goldstein, K., and Scherer, M. "Abstract and Concrete Behaviour." *Psych. Mongr.*, No. 239, 1941.

Graves, R. *The White Goddess*. Faber, London, 1947.

Greene, T. M. "The Problem of Meaning in Music and the Other Arts." *Journ. Aesthetics and Art*, vol. 308, 1947.

Guttmann, E., and Maclay, W. S. "Clinical Observations on Schizophrenic Drawings." *British J. Med. Psychology*, vol. 16, p. 184, 1937.

Guttmann, E. "Artificial Psychoses Produced by Mescalin." *J. Mental Science*, vol. 82, p. 204, 1936.

Halstead, W. C. *Brain and Intelligence*. Univ. Chicago Press, 1947.

Halstead, W. C. "Specialization of Behavioral Function and the Frontal Lobes," Chapter 11 of *The Frontal Lobes*. Williams and Wilkins, Baltimore, 1948.

Head, Sir Henry. *Aphasia and Kindred Disorders of Speech*. Cambridge, 1926.

Henderson and Gillespie. *Textbook of Psychiatry*. Oxford, 1948.

Hull, C. L. *Aptitude Testing*. Harvey & Co., London, 1928.

Hunt, J. McV. "Psychological Experiments with Disordered Persons." *Psychol. Bulletin*, No. 33, 1936.

Hunt, J. McV. *Personality and the Behaviour Disorders* (Chapter 32). Ronald Press, New York, 1944.

Hutton, E., and Bassett, H. "The Effect of Leucotomy on Creative Personality." *J. Mental Science*, vol. 44, p. 332, 1948.

Jaensch, E. R. *Eidetic Imagery*. Kegan Paul, London, 1930.

Jastrow, J. *The House that Freud Built*. Rider, London, 1937.

Jung, C. F. *Psychological Types*. Kegan Paul, London, 1923.

Jung, C. F. "The Psychology of Dementia Praecox." *Nerv. Ment. Dis. Mongr.*, No. 3, 1936.

Kanner, L., and Schilder, P. "Movements in Optic Images and Optic Imagination of Movement." *J. Nerv. & Ment. Dis.*, vol. 72, p. 489, 1930.

Katz, D. *The World of Colour*. Kegan Paul, London, 1935.

Klee, P. *On Modern Art*. Faber, London, 1948.

Kleist, K. *Storungen des Denkens und ihre Hirnpathologischen Grundlagen*. Enke, Stuttgart, 1939.

Kluever, H. "Visual Disturbances after Cerebral Lesions." *Psychol. Bulletin*, vol. 24, p. 316, 1927.

Knauer, A., and Maloney, W. "A Preliminary Note on the Psychic Action of Mescalin." *J. Nerv. & Mental Dis.*, vol. 72, p. 397, 1930.

Koffka, K. *Principles of Gestalt Psychology*. Kegan Paul, London, 1935.

Kretschmer, E. *Medical Psychology*. Kegan Paul, London, 1939.

Lange, J. E., and Eichbaum. *Genie, Irrsinn und Ruhm*, Berlin, 1928.

Lévy-Bruhl, L. *The Soul of the Primitive.* Allen and Unwin, London, 1928.

Lhermitte, J. *L'Image de Notre Corps.* Paris, 1939.

Lowenfeld, V. *Nature of Creative Activity.* Kegan Paul, London, 1939.

Maclay, W. S., and Guttmann, E. "Spontaneous Drawings as an Approach to some Problems in Psychopathology." *Proceed. Roy. Soc. Medicine,* vol. 31, 1937.

Maclay, W. S., and Guttmann, E. "Mescalin Hallucinations in Artists." *Arch. of Neuro. & Psych.,* vol. 45, p. 130, 1941.

Malinowsky, B. *Crime and Custom in Savage Society.* Kegan Paul, London, 1926.

Martin Purdon. "Consciousness and its Disturbances." *The Lancet,* No. 654L–41, 1948–49.

Masserman, J. In—*Modern Trends in Psychological Medicine.* Butterworth, London, 1948.

Masserman, J. *Principles of Dynamic Psychiatry.* Saunders, Philadelphia, 1947.

Maudsley, H. *Natural Causes and Supernatural Seemings.* Thinkers Library, London, 1938.

McIver, R. M. *Society.* Smith, New York, 1931.

Mohr, F. "Über Zeichnungen von Geisteskranken und ihre diagnostische Verwerbarkeit." *J. Psychol. Neurol.,* 1906.

Monakow von. *Die Lokalisation im Grosshirn und der Abbau der Funktion durch kortikale Herde.* Bergmann, Wiesbaden, 1914.

Money-Kyrle, R. *Superstition and Society.* Hogarth Press, London, 1939.

Myers, Sir Charles. "Individual Differences in Listening to Music." *B. J. Psych,* vol. 13, 1923.

Newton, E. *European Painting and Sculpture.* Penguin Books, 1945.

Nicole, E. *Psychopathology.* Baillière & Co., London, 1948.

Noyes, A. *Modern Clinical Psychiatry.* Saunders, Philadelphia, 1939.

Patrick, C. *Archives of Psychology.* New York, No. 178, 1935.

Patrick, C. *Journal of Psychology.* Provincetown, Mass., No. 4, 1937.

Petermann, B. *The Gestalt Theory and the Problem of Configuration.* Kegan Paul, London, 1932.

Petrie, M. *Art and Regeneration.* Elek, London, 1946.

Pötzl, O. "Die optisch-agnostische Störungen." *Handbuch d. Psychiatrie*, Deuticke, Leipzig, 1928.

Prinzhorn, F. *Bildnerei Geisteskranken.* Springer, Berlin, 1922.

Read, H. *Art and Society.* Faber, London, 1945.

Read, H. *Education through Art.* Faber, London, 1947.

Read, H. *The Grass Roots of Art.* Lindsey Drummond, London, 1947.

Reitman, F. "Facial Expression in Schizophrenic Drawings." *J. Mental Sc.*, vol. 85, p. 264, 1939.

Reitman, F. "Lear's Nonsense." *J. of Clinical Psychopathology*, vol. 7, p. 671, 1946.

Reitman, F. "Observations on Personality Changes after Leucotomy." *Journ. Nerv. Ment. Dis.*, No. 6, 105, 1947.

Riddoch, G. "Phantom Limbs and Body Shape." *Brain*, p. 197, 1941.

Roheim, F. "Origin and Function of Culture." *Psycho. Mono.*, 69, New York, 1946.

Rosanoff, A. J. *Manual of Psychiatry.* Wiley, New York, 1938.

Russell, E. S. *Behaviour of Animals.* E. Arnold, London, 1938.

Senden, M. von Raum u. *Gestaltauffassung bei operierten Blinderbornen.* Fischer, Leipzig, 1932.

Schilder, P. *Image and Appearance of the Human Body.* Kegan Paul, London, 1925.

Schilder, P., and Stengel, E. "Asymbolia for Pain." *Arch. Neurol. and Psychiat.*, vol. 25, p. 598, 1931.

Schilder, P. *Mind Perception and Thought.* Columbia Univ. Press, New York, 1942.

Sheldon, W. H. *The Varieties of Human Physique.* Harper, New York, 1940.

Sherrington, Sir Charles. *Man on his Nature.* Cambridge Univ. Press, 1946.

Sigerist, H. E. *Civilization and Disease.* Cornell, New York, 1943.

Spearman, C. *The Abilities of Man.* MacMillan, New York, 1927.

Spearman, C. *Creative Mind.* Nisbet, London, Contemp. Library of Psych., 1930.

Spearman, C. *Psychology down the Ages.* MacMillan, New York, 1937.

Symons, A. J. *The Quest for Corvo.* Penguin, England, 1934.

Thomson, G. *The Factorial Analysis of Human Ability.* Univ. of London Press, 2nd ed., 1946.

Tredgold, A. F. *Textbook of Mental Deficiency.* Baillière, London, 1947.

Valentine, C. W. *Psychology of Early Childhood.* Methuen, London, 1946.

Waddington, C. H. *The Scientific Attitude.* Penguin, 1941.

Wallas, G. *The Art of Thought.* Cape, London, 1926.

Walter, V. J., and Walter, W. G. "The Central Effects of Rhythmic Sensory Stimulation." *Electroenc. and Clinical Neurophys.*, vol. 1, p. 57, 1949.

Wechsler, J. "Partial Cortical Blindness with Preservation of Cortical Vision." *Arch. of Ophthalmology*, 1933.

Weygandt, W. "Zur Frage der pathologischen Kunst." *Z. ges. Neuro. Psych.*, vol. 94, p. 421, 1925.

Wilenski, R. H. *The Modern Movement in Art.* Faber, London, 1945.

Wohlgemuth, A. *A Critical Examination of Psycho-analysis.* Allen and Unwin, London, 1923.

Yenyns, S. *A Background to Chinese Painting.* Sidgwick, London, 1935.

Young, K. *Personality and Problems of Adjustment.* Kegan Paul, London, 1947.

INDEX

Printed and bound by CPI Group (UK) Ltd, Croydon, CR0 4YY

01/11/2024

01782629-0002